# Orthopedic Words and Phrases

A Quick-Reference Guide

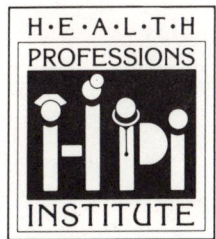

Health Professions Institute • Modesto, California • 1988

## Orthopedic Words and Phrases: A Quick-Reference Guide

© 1988, Health Professions Institute.
All rights reserved.

*Developed by:*

Health Professions Institute
801 15th Street, Suite E
Modesto, California 95354
Telephone (209) 524-4351

*Published by:*

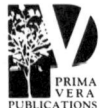

Prima Vera Publications
P. O. Box 801
Modesto, California 95353
Telephone (209) 524-4351
Sally C. Pitman, Editor & Publisher

ISBN 0-934385-12-2

Last digit is the print number: 9 8 7 6 5 4 3 2 1

# Preface

The primary source for **Orthopedic Words and Phrases** is *The SUM Program Orthopedic Transcription Unit* (1988). These educational materials are part of The SUM (**S**ystems **U**nit **M**ethod) Program for training medical transcriptionists, developed by Health Professions Institute.

Numerous transcripts of orthopedic medical and surgical dictation, as well as orthopedic textbooks, scholarly journals, and other references, were carefully reviewed to select more than 13,000 orthopedic words and phrases. The resulting quick-reference guide is a useful reference to medical transcriptionists and other health-care professionals who encounter orthopedic terminology. A list of selected orthopedic references follows page 147.

Many medical transcriptionists contributed to this effort by providing word lists and reviewing transcripts: Shirley Bell, CMT, Carolyn A. Cadigan, CMT, Mary Clithero, Martha Green, CMT, and Charlotte E. Thomas from the Baltimore area; Catherine Gilliam, CMT, Houston; Ruby and Charles Clark, Dallas; Suzanne Taubert, CMT, San Antonio; and from California—Helen Littrell, CMT, Stockton; Bron Taylor, CMT, San Francisco; Donna Taylor, CMT, Santa Ana; and Linda Vourlogianes, Petaluma.

Invaluable assistance in verifying the accuracy of many listings came from Michael A. Ellis, M.D., Baltimore orthopedic surgeon, who generously and patiently answered numerous questions, researched terms, and shared scholarly reference books.

This reference book was produced by the staff and associates of Health Professions Institute: Susan M. Turley, CMT, RN, Curriculum Coordinator, Baltimore; Linda C. Campbell, CMT, Educational Coordinator, Modesto; Vera Pyle, CMT, Consulting Editor, San Francisco; and John H. Dirckx, M.D., Medical Consultant, Dayton, Ohio.

Our warmest gratitude to all.

Sally C. Pitman, CMT, MA
Editor & Publisher

# How To Use This Book

The orthopedic words and phrases in this reference are listed alphabetically and are extensively cross-referenced. An eponymic title may be located alphabetically as well as under the item that it modifies. For example, *Schmeisser spica cast* may be found under both *Schmeisser* and under the main entry *cast*.

Selected medications used frequently in orthopedic medicine and surgery are not listed alphabetically but are located under the main entry *medications*.

To minimize unnecessary duplications, many subentries are combined under one main entry. For example, an orthopedic operation may be referred to as a technique or procedure; however, all techniques and procedures are combined under the main entry *operation*.

A few main entries are listed below.

| | |
|---|---|
| apparatus | medications |
| approach | nail |
| bandage | operation |
| brace | orthosis |
| cast | osteotome |
| classification | osteotomy |
| cup | pin |
| deformity | plate |
| device | position |
| disease | prosthesis |
| dislocation | reamer |
| dressing | reflex |
| drill | retractor |
| elevator | saw |
| fracture | screw |
| frame | sign |
| gait | splint |
| graft | suture |
| guide | syndrome |
| incision | system |
| joint | test |
| ligament | traction |
| maneuver | view |

# Orthopedic Words and Phrases

# A, a

AAA (diagnostic arthroscopy, operative arthroscopy, and possible operative arthrotomy)
AAOS (American Academy of Orthopaedic Surgeons)
A1, A2, A3, A4 pulley
abate, abated, abatement
Abbott-Fisher-Lucas arthrodesis
Abbott-Gill epiphyseal plate exposure
Abbott-Lucas shoulder operation
ABD (abdominal) pad; dressing
abduct, abductor, abduction
abductor digiti minimi manus musculus
abductor digiti minimi pedis musculus
abductor digiti quinti (ADQ)
abet, abetted, abetting
ablation, surgical
ABOS (American Board of Orthopaedic Surgery)
abrader, cartilage
abrasions and contusions
abscess
   Brodie
   collar button
   intraosseous
   subungual
abut, abutted, abutment
AC (acromioclavicular) joint; separation
accessory portion
acclivity
Ace-Colles frame technique
Ace-Fischer external fixator
Ace Unifix fixation device
Ace wrap
acetabular cup (see *cup*)
acetabulectomy
acetabuloplasty
acetabulum, acetabula, acetabular
acetabulum, deep-shelled
ache, aches, achy
acheiria
Achilles tendon lengthening; shortening
Achillis, tendo
achillorrhaphy
achillotenotomy
achondroplasia
achondroplastic dwarfism
ACL (anterior cruciate ligament) repair
acorn, Midas Rex
Acrel ganglion
acrocephalosyndactylism
acrocephalosyndactyly
acromioclavicular
acromionectomy, Armstrong
acromioplasty
   anterior
   McLaughlin
   Neer
acropachy
activities of daily living (ADLs)
ACU-derm wound dressing
ACU-dyne antiseptic
Acufex arthroscopic instruments
Acumeter
adactyly (adactylia)
Adam and Eve splint
adamantinoma
Adamkiewicz, artery of
Adams procedure; saw; splint

adapter
  chuck
  collet screwdriver
  French
  Hudson chuck
  Jacobs chuck
  Lloyd
  Trinkle chuck
Adaptic dressing; gauze; packing
Addis test
adduct, adduction
adduction to neutral
adductor magnus
adductor tendon and lateral capsular release
adductor tenotomy and obturator neurectomy (ATON)
adhesion
  capsular
  fibrous
adhesive (see also *cement*)
  APR cement fixation
  Aron Alpha
  Biobrane
  Coverlet
  cyanoacrylate
  Histoacryl glue
  Implast
  ligand
  medical
  methyl methacrylate
  Simplex cement
  Superglue
  Surfit
adhesive capsulitis
adipose tissue
Adkins arthrodesis; spinal fusion
ADLs (activities of daily living)
ADQ (abductor digiti quinti)
Adson bur; chisel; drill; rongeur; sign
advancement, tendon
advancer
adventitia, adventitial, adventitious
AE (above-elbow) amputation
aerate, aerated, aeration
aerobe, aerobic

Aeroplast dressing
Aesculap-PM noncemented femoral prosthesis
AFI total hip replacement prosthesis
AFO (ankle-foot orthosis)
A-frame orthosis
agenesis, agenetic
AGE (angle of greatest extension)
AGF (angle of greatest flexion)
Agnew splint
Ahern trochanteric debridement
AHSC (Arizona Health Science Center) elbow prosthesis
Aicardi syndrome
AIM CPM (continuous passive motion)
Ainsworth modification of Massie nail
Air-Dyne bicycle
Aitken femoral deficiency
AK (above-knee) amputation (AKA)
Akin bunionectomy; osteotomy
ala, alar
Alanson amputation
Albee-Compere fracture table
Albers-Schönberg disease
Albright-McCune-Sternberg syndrome
alert and oriented x 3 (to person, place, and time)
Alexander-Farabeuf periosteotome
Alexian Brothers overhead frame
align, aligned, alignment
alignment
  anatomic
  poor
  rotational
alignment of fracture fragments
Alimed insert
Alivium implant metal
Allan open reduction of calcaneal fracture
Allen maneuver; sign; test; wrench
Allender vertical laminar flow room
Allis clamps; forceps; sign
Allman classification of acromio-clavicular injury
allogenic bone graft
allograft, bone

*Aircast* (handwritten)

allograft transplantation
alloy
  cobalt-chromium
  stainless steel
Alumafoam splint
aluminum oxide ceramic coating
alveolar rhabdomyosarcoma
amalgam
AMBI hip screw
ambidextrous
ambifixation
ambulate with assistance
ambulatory status
AMC total wrist prosthesis
amelia
American Academy of Orthopaedic Surgeons (AAOS)
American Board of Orthopaedic Surgery (ABOS)
American Seating Access-O-Matic bed
Amigo mechanical wheelchair
AML (amyotrophic lateral sclerosis)
AML hip prosthesis
AML Tang femoral prosthesis
Amoss sign
amphiarthrosis
amputation
  above-elbow (AE)
  above-knee (AK)
  Alanson
  Beclard
  below-knee (BK)
  Berger interscapular
  Bier
  Boyd ankle
  Bunge
  Burgess below-knee
  Callander
  chop
  Chopart
  closed flap
  fishmouth
  guillotine (chop)
  index ray
  interinnominoabdominal
  interphalangeal

amputation *(cont.)*
  Jaboulay
  Lisfranc
  midthigh
  Pirogoff
  ray
  Syme
  transcarpal
amputation stump
amputee
Amspacher-Messenbaugh technique
Amstutz-Wilson osteotomy
amyloid
amyoplasia congenita
amyotonia congenita
amyotrophic lateral sclerosis (AML)
ANA (antinuclear antibody) test
anaerobe, anaerobic
anal wink
analogous
analysis, gait
Anametric total knee system
anastomosis, Riche-Canieu
anatomic snuffbox
anchor plate; splint
anconeus, anconeal, anconoid
Anderson splint; traction
Anderson-D'Alonzo classification
Anderson-Fowler procedure
Anderson-Green growth prediction
Anderson-Hutchins tibial fracture
Andersson hip status system
Andrews iliotibial band reconstruction
anesthesia, anesthetic
  axillary block
  Bier block
  epidural
  general
  general endotracheal
  inhalation, inhalant
  intrathecal
  local standby
  peripheral nerve block
  spinal
  supraclavicular brachial block
  tactile

anesthesia *(cont.)*
    thermal
aneurysmal bone cyst
Anghelescu sign
angiofibroblastic proliferation
angiogram, biplane
angiolipoma
angiosarcoma
angle
    acetabular
    acromial
    Baumann
    Böhler calcaneal
    Böhler lumbosacral
    carrying
    CE (capital epiphysis)
    Citelli
    Codman
    costolumbar
    costosternal
    costovertebral
    Drennan metaphyseal-epiphyseal
    first-fifth intermetatarsal
    first-second intermetatarsal
    hallux valgus
    hallux valgus interphalangeus
    Hilgenreiner
    increased carrying
    intermetatarsal
    Kite
    lumbosacral joint
    Merchant
    metaphyseal-epiphyseal
    Mikulicz
    neck shaft
    Pauwels
    pelvic femoral
    Q
    sacrohorizontal
    sacrovertebral
    set
    sulcus
    talocalcaneal
    talometatarsal
    tibiofemoral (TFA)
    valgus

angle *(cont.)*
    Wiberg
    Wiltze
angle of greatest extension (AGE)
angle of greatest flexion (AGF)
angulation, anterior
ankle mortise
ankylodactyly
ankylosing spondylitis
ankylosis
    bony
    extracapsular
    false
    fibrous
    intracapsular
    ligamentous
    spurious
anlage a priori
anlage, cartilaginous
anneal, annealed
annulotomy
annulus (also anulus)
annulus fibrosus
anode
anomalous insertion
anomaly, congenital
Anspach cement eater
Anspach power drill; reamer
antalgic gait
antebrachial fascia
antecubital fossa
anteflexion
anterior cruciate instability with pivot
    shift
anterior superior iliac spine (ASIS)
anteroposterior (AP)
anteversion
    neutral
    Magilligan technique for measuring
anteversion determination, Budin-
    Chandler
antibiotic and saline solution
antibiotic-impregnated polymethyl
    methacrylate (PMMA)
antiembolic stockings, Orthawear
anti-inflammatory drug (medication)

antimalarial
antinuclear antibody (ANA) test
antiseptic, ACU-dyne
antistreptolysin (ASO) titer
anulus (annulus)
anvil sign
AO nail; plate; screw; technique
AP (anteroposterior)
A-P cutter
APB (abductor pollicis brevis)
Apert disease; syndrome
aperture
aphalangia
APL (abductor pollicis longus)
Apley grinding test
apodia
aponeurectomy
aponeurorrhaphy
aponeurosis, aponeurotic
aponeurotomy
apophysis, apophyseal
apophysitis
apparatus (also called *device*)
  Ace-Fischer external fixator
  Ace Unifix fixation
  adjustable aiming
  Anderson leg lengthening
  AO compression; contouring
  Axer compression
  Bassett electrical stimulation
  body-powered prosthetic
  Bovie electrocautery
  Calandruccio triangular
    compression
  Cameron fracture
  Charnley centering
  collapsible internal fixation
  compression screw-plate
  coracoclavicular fixation
  coring
  CPM
  Day fixation
  Denham external fixation
  Deyerle fixation
  DeWald spinal
  driver tunnel locator

apparatus *(cont.)*
  Dwyer-Wickham electrical
    stimulation
  EBI (electronic bone stimulation)
  electrocautery
  external fixation
  external skeletal fixation
  fixating
  four-bar external fixation
  Fox internal fixation
  Giliberty
  halo-pelvic distraction
  halo vest
  Hare
  Hoffman external fixation
  Hoffman-Vidal external fixation
  Ilizarov
  internal fixation
  Kronner external fixation
  leg-holding
  Müller compression
  nail-bending
  nail-plate
  Nauth traction
  Neufeld
  Orthofix
  Parham-Martin fracture
  Quengel
  Rancho anklet foot control
  Redi-Trac traction
  Rezaian external fixation
  Richards lag screw
  rod-mounted targeting
  Roger Anderson external fixation
  snap-fit
  Southwick pin-holding
  Sutter-CPM knee
  Telectronics electrical stimulation
  Vidal-Ardrey modified Hoffman
    external fixation device
  Volkov-Oganesian external fixation
  Wagner external fixation
  Wagner leg-lengthening
  Wagner-Schanz screw
  Zickel medullary
  Zickel supracondylar fixation

apparatus *(cont.)*
　Zimmer electrical stimulation
appendicular
appliance (see *apparatus*)
application of traction device
apposing articular surfaces
apposition
approach (see also *incision; operation*)
　Abbott knee
　Abbott-Lucas shoulder
　Bailey-Badgley anterior cervical
　Banks-Laufman
　Bennett posterior shoulder
　Boyd
　Brackett-Osgood knee
　Broomhead
　Brown knee
　Bruser knee
　Bryan-Morrey elbow
　Callahan
　Campbell elbow
　Campbell posterior shoulder
　Carnesale hip
　Cave hip; knee
　Cloward cervical disk
　Codman saber-cut shoulder
　Colonna-Ralston ankle
　Coonse-Adam knee
　Cubbins shoulder
　Darrach-McLaughlin
　deltoid-splitting shoulder
　Fahey
　Gatellier-Chastang ankle
　Gibson
　Guleke-Stookey
　Harmon shoulder; cervical
　Henderson
　Henry radial
　Howorth
　Kelikian
　Klein
　Kocher lateral J
　Koenig-Schaefer
　Ludloff
　McWhorter posterior shoulder
　Molesworth-Campbell elbow

approach *(cont.)*
　Moore
　Ollier arthrodesis
　posterolateral
　Roos
　Rowe posterior shoulder
　saber-cut
　Smith-Petersen
　Smith-Robinson cervical disk
　Southwick-Robinson cervical
　split patellar
　sternal-splitting
　Swedish
　Thompson posterior radial
　Wadsworth elbow
　Watson-Jones
　Wiltberger anterior cervical
　Yee posterior shoulder
APR cement fixation
apraxia, apraxic
APRL (Army Prosthetics Research
　Laboratory) prosthesis
apron, quadriceps
Aquaphor gauze dressing
Aquaplast splint
arachnodactyly
arachnoid
Arafiles elbow arthrodesis; prosthesis
arc of motion
arcade of Frohse; Struthers
arch cookie
arch, Hillock
arch support
　plantar
　Plastizote
　Whitman
architecture, bony
arcuate complex
Arizona leg support
arm
　abductor lever
　flail
　linebacker's
　outrigger
　tackler's
　Utah artificial

arm board, Flexisplint flexed
arm cuff
Armistead technique
Armstrong acromionectomy
Army bone gouge; osteotome
Arnold lumbar brace
Arnold-Chiari syndrome
AROM (active range of motion)
Aron Alpha adhesive
arrest, epiphyseal
arthralgia
arthrectomy
arthrempyesis
Arthrex arthroscopy instruments
arthritis, arthritides
  allergenic
  Charcot
  degenerative
  gonococcal
  gouty
  juvenile rheumatoid (JRA)
  Marie-Strümpell
  osteoarthritis
  pauciarticular
  polyarticular
  psoriatic
  rheumatoid
  septic
  suppurative
  traumatic
arthrocele
arthrocentesis
arthrochalasis
arthrochondritis
arthroclasia
arthrodesis (see *operation*)
  compression
  cone
  hindfoot
  intra-articular
  midfoot
  pan-talar
  sliding
  transmalleolar ankle
  triple
arthrodysplasia

arthroendoscopy
arthroereisis
arthrofibrosis
arthrogram
arthrography
  Broström-Gordon
  double-contrast
  Gordon-Broström single-contrast
arthrogryposis multiplex congenita
arthrokatadysis
arthrokleisis
arthrolith
Arthro-Lok blade
arthrolysis
arthromeningitis
arthrometer, stress-testing
arthroncus
arthroneuralgia
arthronosos
arthro-onychodysplasia
arthrophyma
arthrophyte
arthroplasty (see *operation*)
  abrasion
  capitellocondylar total elbow
  cemented total hip
  constrained ankle
  cuff-tear
  cup
  fascial
  interpositional elbow
  modified mold and surface replacement
  monospherical total shoulder
  surface replacement
  total articular resurfacing (TARA)
  triaxial total elbow
Arthropor cup prosthesis; pad
arthropyosis
arthrorheumatism
arthroscope
  angled
  Dyonics
  Eagle straight-ahead
  Storz oblique
  Stryker viewing

arthroscope *(cont.)*
    Wolf
arthroscopic examination
arthroscopy
    diagnostic and operative
    Gilquist
arthrosis
arthrosynovitis
arthrotome
arthrotomy (see *operation*)
arthroxerosis
arthroxesis
articular fragment
articular surfaces
    apposing
    contiguous
articulating bone ends
articulation
    acromioclavicular
    atlantoaxial
    calcaneocuboid
    carpometacarpal
    condylar
    humeroradial
    humeroulnar
    intercarpal
    intermetacarpal
    interphalangeal
    metacarpophalangeal
    patellofemoral
    radiocarpal
    radioulnar
    scapuloclavicular
    subtalar
    talocalcaneonavicular
    tarsometatarsal
    tibiofibular
artifact, artifactual
artificial limb, Utah
Asch forceps; splint
ASE (axilla, shoulder, elbow) bandage
aseptic fashion
aseptic felon (herpetic whitlow)
Ashhurst splint
Ashworth implant arthroplasty
ASIF chisel; plate; screw; technique

ASIS (anterior superior iliac spine)
Asnis cannulated screw
ASO (antistreptolysin O) titer
aspiration
    bone marrow
    joint
assay, radioisotope clearance
astasia
asterixis
asthenia, asthenic
ASTM designation of Biophase
astragalectomy
astragalus, aviator's
asymmetry, asymmetric, asymmetrical
asynergia, asynergic
Atasoy triangular advancement flap
Atasoy V-Y technique
ataxia
    equilibratory
    Friedreich
    Greenfield classification
        of spinocerebellar
    locomotor
Aten olecranon screw
athetosis, athetotic, athetoid
Atkin epiphyseal fracture
Atlanta brace orthosis
atlantoaxial
atlanto-occipital fusion; junction
atlanto-odontoid
atlas (C1, first cervical vertebra)
ATON (adductor tenotomy and
    obturator neurectomy)
atony (atonia)
atraumatic
atretic
atrophic, atrophied
atrophy
    disuse
    Duchenne muscular
    muscle
    quadriceps
    Sudeck
attachment
    capsular
    fibrous

attachment *(cont.)*
   ligamentous
   Pearson
   tendinous
Attenborough knee prosthesis
attenuate, attenuated, attenuating
attenuation (attrition) of tendons
Atton disease
Aufranc modification of Smith-Petersen cup
Aufranc-Cobra hip prosthesis
Aufranc-Turner hip prosthesis
auger
Augustine boat nail
Austin bunionectomy
Austin Moore hip prosthesis
Autoflex II CPM unit
autofusion
autogenous bone graft
autograft, free revascularized
autologous blood transfusion
Autophor ceramic hip prosthesis
autosomal
avascular necrosis (AVN)
Averett hip prosthesis
aviator's astragalus
Avila technique
avulse, avulsed, avulsion
avulsion of nail plate
awl
   Aufranc
   bone
   curved
   DePuy
   Ender
   square-shaped
   Zuelzer
Axer-Clark procedure
Axer varus derotational osteotomy
axial loading of spine
axillary block anesthesia
axis (C2, second cervical vertebra)
axis
   anatomic
   flexion-extension
   long

axis *(cont.)*
   longitudinal
   mechanical
   weightbearing
axle lock and bumper
axonotmesis
azotemic osteodystrophy

# B, b

B. burgdorferi titer for Lyme disease
Babinski reflex; sign
Babinski-Fröhlich syndrome
bacitracin solution
Baciu-Filibiu dowel ankle arthrodesis
back crease
backache
Backhaus towel forceps
Bacon raspatory
Badgley resection of iliac wing
Bagby angled compression plate
Bahler hinge
bail-lock knee joint
Bailey-Badgley cervical spine fusion
Bailey-Dubow technique
Bailey-Gigli saw guide
Baker lateral semitendinosus transfer
Baker-Hill osteotomy
Balacescu-Golden technique
Balkan fracture frame; splint
ball-and-socket joint
ball bearing, Steinmann pin with
ball, cold-weld femoral
Ballenger periosteotome
Ballenger-Hajek chisel
ballotable
ballottement of patella
balsa wood filler block

band
  AO tension
  calf
  fascial
  iliotibial (IT)
  lateral
  Parham-Martin
  scar
bandage (see also *dressing*)
  Ace adherent
  ASE (axilla, shoulder, elbow)
  Barton
  capeline
  compression
  cotton elastic
  cravat
  demigauntlet
  Desault
  Elastoplast
  Esmarch
  Flex-Foam
  Flex-Master
  gauntlet
  Gibney
  Gibson
  gum rubber Martin
  Hamilton
  Helenca
  Heliodorus
  Hippocrates
  Hueter
  immobilizing
  Kling elastic
  Martin sheet rubber
  Ortho-Trac
  Ortho-Vent
  PRN
  Pavlik
  plaster of Paris (POP)
  Redigrip pressure
  replantation
  restrictive
  Ribble
  Richet
  Sayre
  scultetus

bandage *(cont.)*
  sling-and-swath
  spica
  spiral
  starch
  stockinette
  Velpeau
  Webril
Bandi procedure
Bankart procedure for shoulder dislocation
Bankart-Putti-Platt operation
Banks-Laufman approach; technique
bantenadesis
bar (see also *splint*)
  bony
  Denis Browne (DB)
  Gerster traction
  intramedullary
  Livingston intramedullary
  lumbrical
  metatarsal flatfoot
  opponens
  patellar
  spacer
  Stephen spreader
  Thornton
  unsegmented vertebral
barber chair position
barbotage
Bard-Parker scalpel; blade
Barlow maneuver; sign; splint; test
Barr-Record ankle arthrodesis
Barrasso-Wile-Gage arthrodesis
Barsky procedure; technique
Bartlett nail fold excision
Barton-Cone tong traction
base of fingernail
base, Dycal
baseball elbow
Basile screw
basioccipital
basket, shovel-nose Schutte
Bassett electrical stimulation device
Basswood splint

Batch-Spittler-McFaddin knee
   disarticulation
Batchelor-Brown arthrodesis
Bateman UPF (universal proximal
   femur) prosthesis
bath
   contrast
   paraffin (PB)
   whirlpool
battledore incision
Bauer-Tondra-Trusler technique
Baumann angle
Baumgard-Schwartz tennis elbow
   technique
Bavarian splint
Baylor splint
bayonet position of fracture
beach chair position
bead, targeting
beaking of head of talus
Beall-Webel-Bailey technique
beanbag
Beath needle; pin; view
Beaver-DeBakey blades
Bebax shoe for forefoot deformity
Bechtol acetabular component
Beckenbaugh technique
Becker muscular dystrophy
Beckman retractor
Beclard amputation
Becton technique
bed
   American Seating Access-O-Matic
   Borg-Warner orthopedic
   Carrom orthopedic
   CircOlectric
   DMI orthopedic
   Foster
   fracture
   Gatch
   gatched
   Goodman orthopedic
   Hausted orthopedic
   Hill-Rom orthopedic
   Hollywood
   Inland Super Multi-Hite orthopedic

bed *(cont.)*
   Inter-Royal frame orthopedic
   Joerns orthopedic
   nail
   Simmons Multi-Matic orthopedic
   Simmons Vari-Hite orthopedic
   Smith-Davis Converta-Hite
   Superior Sleeprite Hi-Lo orthopedic
   Ultra-Flex orthopedic
bed cradle
bed rest
Beeson cast spreader
Beevor sign
Bekhterev-Mendel reflex
Bell-Dally cervical dislocation
Bell-Tawse open reduction technique
Bellemore-Barrett-Middleton-Scougall-
   Whiteway technique
belly, muscle
belt
   Posey
   Silesian
   waist suspension
   Zim-Zap rib
Bence Jones protein
bench examination
bender
   French rod
   Rush
Bendixen-Kirschner traction
Bennett posterior shoulder approach
Berger interscapular amputation
Berman-Gartland metatarsal osteotomy
Berman-Moorhead metal locator
Bermuda spica cast
Berndt hip ruler
Berstein cast table
Betadine soak; scrub solution
Bethesda bone
Bethune periosteal elevator
bevel, beveled, beveling
Bevin shoe
Beyer rongeur
B.H. Moore procedure
biceps
   long head of

biceps *(cont.)*
　short head of
　biceps femoris
bicipital tendinitis
Bickel leg holder
Bickel-Moe procedure
bicondylar fracture
bicortical screw
bicycle, Air-Dyne
Bier block anesthesia
bifid
Bigelow
bikini skin incision
Bilos pin
bimalleolar ankle fracture
binder (see also *bandage; dressing*)
　Helenca
　scultetus
binding, biological
Bioclusive dressing
Biofit acetabular prosthesis
Biolox ceramic coating
biomechanics
Biomet prosthesis
Biophase implant metal
Biophase, ASTM designation of
biopsy
　bone marrow
　channel and core
　Dunn
　forage core
Biotex implant metal
bipartite
Bircher-Weber technique
Bishop-Black tendon tucker
Bishop-DeWitt tendon tucker
Bishop-Peter tendon tucker
BKA (below-knee amputation)
Black-Broström staple technique
Blackburn traction
blade (see *knife*)
blade plate (see *plate*)
Blair chisel; elevator
Blair-Brown skin graft
Blair-Morris-Dunn-Hand arthrodesis
blanch, blanched, blanching

Blazina prosthesis
Bleck recession technique
Bledsoe brace
blister of bone
block
　axillary
　balsa wood filler
　bone
　Campbell posterior bone
　cutting
　filler
　Gill posterior bone
　Howard bone
　Inclan posterior bone
　Mikhail bone
　nerve
　peripheral nerve
　regional
　stellate sympathetic ganglion
　Styrofoam filler
blood supply, longitudinal
Bloom splint
Bloom-Raney modification of Smith-
　Robinson technique
Blount-Schmidt Milwaukee brace
Blumensaat line
Blumer shelf
Blundell Jones technique
BMP (bone marrow pressure)
board
　spinal
　Yucca
Bock knee prosthesis
body, bodies
　intra-articular
　loose
　rice
　vertebral
body mechanics
Boeck sarcoid
boggy synovitis
Böhler (Boehler) angle
Böhler-Braun splint
Böhler-Steinmann pin holder
Bohlman cervical vertebrectomy
Boies forceps

bolster
  abduction
  rubber
bolt
  Barr
  cannulated
  Fenton
  fixation
  Harris
  Holt
  Moreira
  tibial
  Webb stove
  Zimmer tibia
bolt cutter
bolus, cotton
Bombelli-Mathys-Morscher hip prosthesis
Bond splint
bone
  accessory
  Bethesda
  brittle
  cancellous
  chalky
  compact
  cortical
  cuneiform
  eburnated
  endochondral
  flat
  fragmental
  freeze-dried
  heterotopic
  infected
  ivory
  lamellar
  lamellated
  long
  long axis of
  luxated
  marble
  nonlamellated
  osteonal
  osteoporotic
  pagetoid

bone *(cont.)*
  Pirie
  primitive
  raw
  rider's
  rudimentary
  semilunar
  sesamoid
  short
  spongy
  subchondral
  woven
bone age, Greulich and Pyle
bone bank
bone block (see *block*)
bone chip
bone cutter, Horsley
bone debris
bone density
bone ends
bone fragments
bone graft (see *graft*)
bone graft incorporation
bonelet
bone marrow pressure (BMP)
bonemeal tablet
bone remodeling
bone resurfacing
bone scan (see *scan*)
bone skid, Murphy-Lane
bone spreader, Blount
bone stock, poor
bone substance
bone wax, Horsley
Bonfiglio modification of Phemister technique
bony necrosis and destruction
boot
  Bunny
  cast
  gelatin compression
  Gibney
  moon
  rocker
  Unna
  Unna's paste

| boot | 20 | brace |
|---|---|---|

boot *(cont.)*
    Wilke
boot wrap, Unna
Boplant surgibone
Bora operation
borer
    bone
    cork
Borg-Warner orthopedic bed
Borggreve-Hall technique
Bose nail fold excision
boss, bossing
bosselated, bosselation
Boston thoracic brace
Bosworth femoroischial arthrodesis
botryoid sarcoma
Bouchard node
Bouge needle
bouncing, ligamentous
boutonnière deformity
Bovie electrocautery apparatus
bow
    Böhler
    Kirschner wire
    posterior
    traction
Bowden cable suspension system
bowed legs
Bowen-Grover meniscotome
Bowlby splint
bowleg (genu varum)
Bowlly splint
Bowman angle
box
    anatomic snuffbox
    high-toe
Boyd-Anderson biceps tendon repair
Boyd-Bosworth procedure
Boyd-Griffin classification
Boyd-McLeod procedure
Boyd-Sisk posterior capsulorrhaphy
Boyes brachioradialis transfer
Bozzini light conductor
brace (see also *bar; orthosis; splint*)
    Arnold lumbar
    back

brace *(cont.)*
    Bledsoe
    Blount-Schmidt Milwaukee
    boot
    Boston thoracic
    bowleg
    cable twister
    caliper
    Callender derotational
    Can Am
    carpenter's
    cast
    Castiglia ankle
    chairback
    Charnley
    CHH cervical
    Chopart
    clam-shell
    Cole hyperextension
    controlled-motion
    Cook walking
    cowhorn
    CTI
    Dennyson cervical
    dial-lock
    Don Joy knee
    drop-lock knee
    drop foot
    dynamic abduction
    Florida cervical
    footdrop
    49er knee
    four-point cervical
    four-poster cervical
    Friedman
    Guilford cervical
    Hennessy knee
    Hudson
    hyperextension
    ischial weightbearing
    Jewett hyperextension
    King cervical
    Klengall
    Klenzak spring
    Knight back
    Knight-Taylor thoracic

*Kallassy ankle braces (not Kalessy)*

brace — 21 — Brittain

brace *(cont.)*
  knock-knee
  Kydex
  lacing ankle
  Lenox Hill derotational knee
  long arm
  long leg hinged
  LSU reciprocation-gait orthosis
  lumbar
  Lyman-Smith
  MacCausland lumbar
  Medipedic Multicentric knee
  Milwaukee
  Moon Boot
  Mooney
  Murphy
  neoprene
  Newington
  night
  nonweightbearing
  Oppenheim
  patellar tendon-bearing
  P.C. Williams
  Phelps
  Philadelphia Plastizote cervical
  Pro-8 ankle
  PTS knee
  reamer
  Rolyan tibial fracture
  Saltiel
  Schanz   *Sarmiento*
  scoliosis
  Scottish Rite
  Seton hip
  short arm
  short leg double upright
  snap-lock
  SOMI (sterno-occipital-mandibular
    immobilizer)
  stirrup
  Taylor-Knight
  Teufel
  Thomas
  TLSO (thoracolumbosacral orthosis)
  toe drop
  Toronto

brace *(cont.)*
  Tracker knee
  Trinkle
  UBC (Univ. of British Columbia)
  unilateral calcaneal (UCB)
  Varney acromioclavicular
  Victorian
  walking
  Warm Springs
  Watco
  weightbearing
  Williams
  Yale
  Zimmer reamer
brace/corset, Hoke lumbar
brachialgia
brachioradialis tendon
brachium
Brackett-Osgood-Putti-Abbott
  technique
Bradford fracture frame
Brady leg splint
Brady-Jewett technique
Bragard sign
Brain variation, hip arthroplasty
branch
  motor
  proper digital nerve
Brand tendon transfer technique
Brannon-Wickstrom technique
Brant aluminum splint
Brantigan-Voshell procedure
brassiere, Jobst
Braun shoulder tenotomy
breastbone
Brett-Campbell tibial osteotomy
Breuerton x-ray view of hand
bridge of meniscus
bridging osteophytes
Brigham prosthesis
Brighton electrical stimulation system
brisement
Bristow-Helfet procedure
Bristow-May procedure
British test
Brittain ischiofemoral arthrodesis

broach
  barbed
  drilling
  femoral prosthesis
    Harris
    Mittlemeir
    root canal
    smooth
    Zimmer femoral canal
Brodie abscess; disease
Brooker-Willis nail
Brookes-Jones tendon transfer
Brooks-Jenkins atlantoaxial fusion technique
Brooks-Seddon tendon transfer
Broomhead approach
Brophy periosteal elevator
Broström-Gordon arthrography
Brown knee joint reconstruction
Brown-Séquard syndrome
Brudzinski sign
Bruening-Citelli rongeur
bruisability
Brun bone curet
Brunn plaster shears
Bruser skin incision (knee surgery)
Bryan-Morrey elbow approach
Bryant sign; traction
Buchholz acetabular cup
Buck plug; splint; traction
Buck-Gramcko pollicization
bucket, Denis Browne
Bucky x-ray tray
buddy taping
Budin-Chandler anteversion determination
buffalo hump
Bugg-Boyd technique
bulb, irrigation
bulbus (n.), bulbous (adj.)
bulla, bullae, bullous
bump
  hip
  inion
  runner's
Buncke technique

bundle function
bundle, neurovascular
Bunge amputation
bunionectomy
  Akin
  Austin
  chevron
  DuVries-Mann modified
  Keller
  Kreuscher
  Lapidus
  McBride
  Silver
  tailor's
bunion-hallux valgus complex
bunionette-hallux valgus-splay foot complex
Bunker foot piece
Bunnell drill; splint; stitch
Bunnell modification of Steindler flexorplasty
bur (also *burr*)
  Adson
  Bailey
  bone
  Burwell
  Caparosa
  carbide
  cone
  conical
  crosscut
  Cushing
  cutting
  dental
  high-speed
  Midas Rex
  Ossotome
  power
  Zimmer rotary
bur hole
Burch-Greenwood tendon tucker
Burgess below-knee amputation
Burkhalter modification of Stiles-Bunnell technique
Burnham thumb and finger splint
Burns plate

burr (see *bur)*
Burrows technique
bursa, bursae
  adventitious
  ischiogluteal
  Luschka
  olecranon
  retrocalcaneal
  subacromial
  trochanteric
bursal sac
bursectomy
bursitis
  anserine
  ischial gluteal
  ischiogluteal
  prepatellar
  septic
  Tornwaldt
bursocentesis
bursolith
bursopathy
bursotomy
Burton sign
Burwell bur
bushing, guide
Butler fifth toe operation
button
  Drummond
  Hewson ligament
  padded
  patellar
buttress plate; screw
buttressing
buzz bleeders

## C, c

C-bar on orthosis
C-arm
C-reactive protein
C-spine (cervical spine)
C-washer
C-wire inserter
cable
  Dwyer scoliosis
  twister
Cabot splint
CAD femoral stem prosthesis
Cadenza panty/girdle
Caffey disease
caisson worker's disease
Calandruccio compression apparatus
calcaneal spur pad in shoe
calcaneoclavicular ligament
calcaneocuboid joint
calcaneonavicular coalition
calcaneotibial fusion
calcar, pivot of
calcify, calcified, calcification
calcinosis circumscripta
Calcitite graft material
calcium hydroxyapatite
Caldwell-Coleman flatfoot technique
Caldwell-Durham tendon transfer
caliper
  blunt
  Thomas walking
  Townley femur
  Vernier
  weight-relieving
Callahan extension of cervical injury
Callahan fusion technique
Callander amputation
Callaway test
Calleja exercises
Callender derotation brace
callosity, callosities
callous (adj.), callus (n.)
Calloway test

*Kegel exercises*

callus
  bridging
  florid
  fracture
callus formation
callus weld
Calnan-Nicole prosthesis
Caltagirone chisel
Calve-Perthes disease
Cameron-Haight periosteal elevator
Camitz tendon transfer
Camp corset
Campbell-Akbarnia procedure
Campbell-Goldthwait procedure
Camper chiasma
camptocormia
camptodactyly
Can Am brace
Canadian crutch
Canakis pin
canal
  femoral
  Guyon
  haversian
  intramedullary
  medullary
  Volkmann
Canale osteotomy
canaliculus, canaliculi
cancellectomy
cancellous versus cortical bone
candle wax appearance of bone
cane
  quadrapod
  tripod
cannula
  Acufex double lumen arthroscopic
  arthroscopic
  Dyonics
  inflow
  large bore inflow
  microirrigating
  suprapatellar
cannulated guided hip screw system
Cantelli sign
Caparosa bur; wire crimper

Capener rhachotomy
capillary filling time
capital epiphysis (CE) angle
capitate
capitellocondylar total elbow
  arthroplasty
capitellum
capitular epiphysis
capitulocondylar elbow arthroplasty
Capner splint
capsular imbrication
capsule
  articular
  Gerota
  joint
  metatarsophalangeal joint
  posterolateral
capsulectomy, anterior
capsulitis, adhesive
capsulodesis, Zancolli
capsuloperiosteal envelope
capsuloplasty, Zancolli
capsulorrhaphy (see *operation*)
  medial
  pants-over-vest
  staple
capsulotomy (see *operation*)
  Curtis PIP joint
  dorsal transverse
  dorsolateral and medial
  V
carbide bur
Carceau-Brahms ankle arthrodesis
Cardan screwdriver
Carl P. Jones traction splint
Carnesale-Stewart-Barnes classification
  of hip dislocation
carpal row
carpal tunnel release (CTR)
carpectomy
carpi radialis brevis tendon
carpi radialis longus tendon
carpometacarpal articulation
Carrell fibular substitution technique
Carrell-Girard screw
Carroll-Legg periosteal elevator

*CASH brace*

Carroll 25 cast

Carroll-Smith-Petersen osteotome
Carrom orthopedic bed
Carter pillow; splint
Carter-Rowe view
cartilage
   articular
   patellofemoral groove
   quadrangle
   shelling off of
   triradiate
cartilaginous anlage; cap
cast
   airplane
   arm cylinder
   banjo
   below-knee walking
   below-the-knee
   bent-knee
   Bermuda spica
   bivalved cylinder
   body
   Boston bivalve
   corrective
   Cotrel scoliosis
   cotton
   cottonloader position
   Cutter
   cylinder walking
   Dehne
   double-hip spica
   double spica
   EDF scoliosis
   extension body
   fiberglass
   figure 8 (figure-of-8)
   flexion body
   Fractura Flex
   Frejka
   full-thumb spica
   Gaiter
   gauntlet
   Gelocast
   groin-to-ankle
   Gypsona
   halo
   hanging arm

cast *(cont.)*
   Hexcelite
   hinged cylinder
   hip spica
   Kite clubfoot
   Kite metatarsal
   light
   long arm (LAC)
   long leg (LLC)
   long leg bent-knee
   long leg walking (LLWC)
   Lorenz
   Lovell clubfoot
   MaxCast
   Minerva
   Moe modified Cotrel
   Mooney
   Neufeld
   nonwalking
   O'Donoghue cotton
   one and one-half spica
   one-half spica
   patellar tendon weightbearing
   patellar tendon-bearing (PTB)
   Petrie spica
   plaster of Paris
   polyurethane
   Quengel
   Risser localizer scoliosis
   Risser turnbuckle
   Sarmiento short leg patellar
      tendon-bearing
   Sbarbaro spica
   Schmeisser spica
   scoliosis
   serial wedge
   short arm (SAC)
   short arm fiberglass
   short leg (SLC)
   short leg walking (SLWC)
   shoulder spica
   slipper-type
   spica
   sugar-tong
   three-finger spica
   thumb spica

cast (cont.)
  toe spica
  toe-to-groin
  toe-to-midthigh
  turnbuckle
  univalve
  Velpeau
  walking
  walking boot
  warm-and-form
  wedging
  well leg
  windowed
cast application
castbelt, Posey below-the-knee
cast breaker
  Böhler
  Wolfe-Böhler
cast cover, Dryspell
cast cushion, FB
cast cutter, Redi-Vac
casting, intermittent
cast padding, cotton
cast sock
cast spreader
  Beeson
  Hoffer-Daimler
cast table, Berstein
cast tape
  Scotchcast 2
  TufStuf II
cast walker
  rubber sole
  Sabel
cast wedge, Yancy
cast window
cast with dorsal (or volar) toe plate extension
Castiglia ankle brace
Castle procedure
Castroviejo bladebreaker knife
casts, serial wedged
category, Westin-Turco
Cathcart Orthocentric hip prosthesis
Catterall classification
cauda equina syndrome

causalgia
cautery
  bipolar
  Bovie
  unipolar
Cave-Rowe shoulder dislocation technique
Cavin osteotome
cavity
  joint
  marrow
  saclike
cavovarus deformity
CAWO (closing abductory wedge osteotomy)
CDH (congenital dysplasia, or dislocation, of hip)
CE (capital epiphysis) angle of Wiberg
Cebotome
cell
  multipotential
  myxomatous
  osteogenic
  Schwann
  specialized
  spindle
cellulitis
cement (see also *adhesive*)
  acrylic
  bone
  Ketac
  low-viscosity
  methyl methacrylate
  orthopedic
  Palacos
  pressurization of
  Protoplast
  Surgical Simplex P radiopaque
  Zimmer low-viscosity
cement compactor, acetabular
cement eater
  Anspach
  Zimmer Cibatome
cement removal
cement technique
cemented total hip arthroplasty

| cementless | 27 | chondromalacia |

cementless technique
cementome, Anspach
cementophyte
cephalad
cerclage
cerebral palsy (CP)
    ataxic
    athetoid
    dyskinetic
    flaccid
    spastic
cerebroside reticulocytosis
cerebrospinal fluid (CSF)
Cerva Crane halter
cervical brace (see *brace*)
cervical orthosis (see *orthosis*)
cervical spine (C1 to C7)
cervical support (see *support*)
cervicothoracolumbosacral orthosis
cervicotrochanteric
Chaddock sign
Chamberlain line
chamfer cut
Chance vertebral fracture
Chandler felt collar splint
Chapchal knee arthrodesis
Charcot-Marie-Tooth disease
Charest head frame
charley horse
Charnley hip arthroplasty
Charnley-Houston shoulder arthrodesis
Charnley-Mueller hip prosthesis
Charriere bone saw
Chatfield-Girdlestone splint
Chatzidakis hinged Vitallium implant
Chaves muscle transfer
Chaves-Rapp muscle transfer technique
check socket
cheilectomy
    Garceau
    Mann-Coughlin-DuVries
chemonucleolysis, double-needle
Cherry-Austin drill
chevron laceration
Cheyne periosteal elevator
CHH cervical brace

Chiari innominate osteotomy
chiasma, Camper
Chick fracture table
Chiene test
chilblains
Childress ankle fixation technique
chin-occiput piece
Chinese fingertrap
chiropractor
chisel
    Adson
    Alexander
    ASIF
    Ballenger-Hajek
    Blair
    Bowen
    box
    Brittain
    Caltagirone
    Cinelli-McIndoe
    Cloward
    cold
    Hibbs
    Meyerding
    seating
    Simmons
    Smillie cartilage
    square hollow
    swan-neck
Cho cruciate ligament reconstruction
Cho tendon technique
chondral fragment
chondralgia
chondrectomy
chondritis
chondroblastoma
chondrodysplasia
chondrodystrophia calcificans
chondrodystrophia fetalis
chondroepiphysitis
chondrofibroma
chondrolipoma
chondrolysis
chondroma, juxtacortical
chondromalacia of the patella
chondromalacia patellae

chondromalacic
chondromatosis, synovial
chondrometaplasia
chondromyofibroma
chondromyxofibroma
chondromyxoid fibroma
chondromyxoma
chondromyxosarcoma
chondronecrosis
chondro-osteodystrophy
chondropathology
chondrophyte
chondroplasty, chondroplastic
chondroporosis
chondrosarcoma
    clear cell
    differentiated
    extraskeletal
    mesenchymal
    periosteal
chondrosarcomatosis
chondrosteoma
chondrosternoplasty
chondrotomy
Chopart partial foot prosthesis
chordoma
chorea, Huntington
choreiform
Chrisman-Snook ankle technique
Christensen interlocking nail
Christiansen hip prosthesis
Christmas hemophiliac disease
Christmas tree reamer
chromated catgut suture
chromatolysis
chuck
    hand
    Jacobs
    pin
Chuinard-Peterson ankle arthrodesis
Chvostek sign
cicatrix
Cincinnati incision
Cinelli-McIndoe chisel
Cintor knee prosthesis
CircOlectric bed; frame
circulatory embarrassment
circumference
    calf
    pelvic
Citelli angle
Claiborne external fixator
clamp
    Adair breast
    Allis
    Böhler
    bone-holding
    Boyes muscle
    C
    Charnley compression
    gallbladder
    Harrington hook
    Hoen
    Kelly
    Kern bone
    Kocher
    Lahey
    Lambert-Lowman bone
    Lane bone
    Lewin bone-holding
    Lowman bone
    Martin meniscus
    Mayo
    meniscus
    microvascular
    mosquito
    patellar
    self-retaining
    towel
    Verbrugge
Clancy cruciate ligament reconstruction
Clark transfer technique
classification
    Aitken epiphyseal fracture
    Allman acromioclavicular injury
    acromioclavicular injury
    Anderson-D'Alonzo odontoid fracture
    Boyd-Griffin trochanteric fracture
    Carnesale-Stewart-Barnes hip dislocation

classification *(cont.)*
 Catterall
 Colonna hip fracture
 Delbert hip fracture
 Dickhaut-DeLee discoid meniscus
 Dyck-Lambert
 Essex-Lopresti calcaneal fracture
 Evans intertrochanteric fracture
 Fielding-Magliato subtrochanteric fracture
 Freeman calcaneal fracture
 Frykman radial fracture
 Garden femoral neck fracture
 Gartland supracondylar fracture
 Grantham femur fracture
 Greenfield (spinocerebellar ataxia)
 Gustilio puncture wound
 Hansen fracture
 Hohl tibial condylar fracture
 Holdsworth spinal fracture
 Ingram-Bachynski hip fracture
 Jeffery radial fracture
 Key-Conwell pelvic fracture
 Kilfoyle condylar fracture
 Lauge-Hansen ankle fracture
 Leung thumb loss
 MacNichol-Voutsinas
 Mason radial fracture
 Meyers-McKeever tibial fracture
 Milch elbow fracture
 Neer femur fracture
 Neer shoulder fracture
 Neer-Horowitz humerus fracture
 Newman radial fracture
 O'Brien radial fracture
 Ogden epiphyseal fracture
 O'Rahilly limb deficiency
 Pauwels femoral neck fracture
 Pipkin femoral fracture
 Poland epiphyseal fracture
 Ratliff avascular necrosis
 Riseborough-Radin intercondylar fracture
 Rockwood acromioclavicular injury
 Rowe calcaneal fracture

classification *(cont.)*
 Sage-Salvatore acromioclavicular joint injury
 Saha shoulder muscle
 Sakellarides calcaneal fracture
 Salter epiphyseal fracture
 Salter-Harris epiphyseal fracture
 Seinsheimer femoral fracture
 Shelton femur fracture
 Sorbie calcaneal fracture
 Thompson-Epstein femoral fracture
 Tronzo intertrochanteric fracture
 Vostal radial fracture
 Warren-Marshall
 Wassel thumb duplication
 Watanabe discoid meniscus
 Watson-Jones tibial fracture
 Wiberg (patella)
 Wilkins radial fracture
 Winquist-Hansen femoral fracture
 Zlotsky-Ballard acromioclavicular injury
clavicectomy
clavicotomy
clavipectoral fascia
clawfoot deformity
clawhand deformity
clawtoe deformity
Clayton forefoot arthroplasty
Clayton-Fowler technique
clearance, radioactive xenon
Cleeman sign
cleft, interinnominoabdominal
cleidocranial dysostosis
Cleland ligament in the hand
Cleveland-Bosworth-Thompson technique
click, clicking
click, hip
clinodactyly
clock, shoulder
clonus
 drawn ankle
 three-beat
closed reduction, internal fixation

closing abductory wedge osteotomy (CAWO)
closing wedge manipulation and reapplication of plaster
closure
  delayed
  epiphyseal
  primary
  secondary
cloverleaf Küntscher nail
Cloward anterior spinal fusion
Cloward chisel; drill; hammer
clubbing of fingers, toes
clubfoot splint, Denis Browne
clubhand
Co-Cr-Mo (cobalt-chromium-molybdenum) alloy implant metal
Co-Cr-W-Ni (cobalt-chromium-tungsten-nickel) alloy implant metal
coagulase negative
coagulase positive
coapt, coapted, coaptation
Coballoy implant metal
cobalt-chromium alloy
Coban elastic dressing; wrap
Cobb attachment for Albee-Compere fracture table
Cobb scoliosis measuring technique
coccygeal spine (coccyx)
coccygectomy
coccygodynia
coccygotomy
coccyodynia (see *coccygodynia*)
coccyx (coccygeal spine)
cock-up hand splint
Codivilla tendon lengthening technique
Codman angle; drill; exercises
Cofield shoulder prosthesis
cogwheel gait
Colclough laminectomy rongeur
cold-weld femoral ball; prosthesis
Cole fracture frame
Coleman flatfoot technique
collagen, microcrystalline
collar
  cervical

collar *(cont.)*
  Forrester-Brown
  Lewin
  myocervical
  periosteal bone
  Philadelphia
  Plastizote cervical
  Schanz
  serpentine foam
  Thomas
collar bone
collateral circulation
Colles' fracture; splint
collet screwdriver adapter
Collis broken femoral stem technique
Collison drill; plate; screw
Colonna-Ralston ankle approach
Coltart fracture technique
Comforfoam splint
comminuted intra-articular fracture
commissural myelorrhaphy
Comolli sign
compacter, acetabular cement
compartment
  anterior
  deep posterior
  lateral
  medial
  patellofemoral
  posterior
  posterolateral
  posteromedial
  superficial posterior
Compartmental II knee prosthesis
compensatory wedge
Compere-Thompson arthrodesis
complex
  arcuate
  bunionette-hallux valgus-splay foot
  bunion-hallux valgus
  fabellofibular
  Ghon-Sachs
  hallux valgus-metatarsus primus varus
component (see also *prosthesis*)
  acetabular

component (cont.)
   AML trial hip
   Amstutz femoral
   Aufranc-Turner femoral
   Bechtol acetabular
   Bombelli-Morscher femoral
   Charnley narrow stem;
     standard stem
   cobra-design femoral
   DePuy trispiked acetabular
   glenoid
   humeral
   metal-backed acetabular
   Neer II humeral
   prosthesis
   Tri-Con
   trial femoral
component trial
compression apparatus, Calandruccio
Compton clavicle pin
Conaxial ankle prosthesis
concave, concavity
concretion
concurrent
condyle, condylar
condylectomy
condylocephalic nailing
condylotomy
Cone ring curet
confluent
Conform dressing
congenital dysplasia of the hip (CDH)
congenital intercalary limb absence
congenital laxity of ligament
congenital terminal limb absence
congestion, flap
Conley pin
Conray contrast media
conservative management
consolidation
constant touch perception
constriction, hourglass
contiguous articular surfaces
continuity
Contour internal prosthesis
contour, Wiberg type II patellar

contract, contracted, contraction
contracture
   Dupuytren
   fixed flexion
   flexion
   ischemic
   muscle
   soft tissue
   Volkmann ischemic
   web
contralateral sign
contrast media
contrecoup injury
control
   Dupaco knee
   exsanguination tourniquet
   image
   swing phase
contusion, hip
convex, convexity
Cook walking brace
cookie
   arch
   navicular shoe
   scaphoid shoe
   shoe
cookie cutter
Coonrad hinge prosthesis
Coonse-Adams technique
Coopernail sign
coracoacromial process
coracoclavicular fixation device
coracohumeral ligament
coracoid process
cord compression
cord portion
cord
   heel
   pretendinous
cordlike structure
cordotomy
corn
   end
   plantar
   web
Cornelia de Lange syndrome

coronoid process
correction, scoliosis
corset
   Camp
   elastic ankle
   Kampe
   leather ankle
   lumbosacral
cortex, cortices
cortex, femoral
cortical desmoid
cortical versus cancellous bone
corticotomy of proximal tibia
Coryllos-Doyen periosteal elevator
cosmesis, poor
cosmetically and functionally
   normal
costectomy
costochondral junction of ribs
costochondritis
costosternal angle
costotransversectomy technique
costovertebral angle (CVA) tenderness
Cotrel scoliosis
Cotrel-Dubousset spinal instrument
Cottle osteotome; rasp; saw
Cotton ankle fracture
cottonloader position cast
cottonoid patty
Couch-Derosa-Throop transfer
   technique
counter
   extended medial shoe
   Geiger
   heel
counterbore, cloverleaf
countersink, countersunk
Coventry femoral osteotomy
Cover-Roll adhesive gauze
coxa adducta
coxa brevis
coxa magna
coxa plana
coxa valga
coxa vara
coxa vara luxans

coxarthria
coxarthritis
coxarthropathy
coxarthrosis
coxitis
Cozen test
Cozen-Brockway Z-plasty
CP (cerebral palsy)
CPM (continuous passive motion)
CPM device, machine
crabmeat-like appearance
Cracchiolo forefoot arthroplasty
cracking of joint
Craig splint
Cramer wire splint
cramp, muscle
Crane osteotome
cranial nerves II-XII intact
Crawford low lithotomy crutches
Crawford-Adams cup arthroplasty
creaking
crease
   alar
   back
   infragluteal
   palmar
   popliteal
   skin
   thenar
Crego femoral osteotomy
Crego-McCarroll traction
crepitant, crepitation
crepitation, patellofemoral
crepitus, bony
crescent-shaped fibrocartilaginous disk
crescentic rupture
crest, iliac
Crile head traction
crista
criteria, Insall
crossunion
Crowe pilot point
crown
   Adaptic
   Unitek steel
cruciate fashion

cruciform screwdriver
crural fascia
crutch walking, nonweightbearing
crutches
   Canadian
   Crawford low lithotomy
   Lofstrand
   weightbearing
Crutchfield-Raney tongs
cryotherapy, liquid nitrogen
cryptotic medial border
crystal
   urate
   uric acid
crystalloid
CSF (cerebrospinal fluid)
CT (computerized tomographic) scan
CTI brace — *see brace*
CTLSO (cervicothoracolumbosacral orthosis)
CTR (carpal tunnel release)
Cubbins shoulder dislocation technique
cubital tunnel syndrome
cubitus valgus
cubitus varus
cuff
   arm
   pneumatic tourniquet
   rotator
   thigh
cuff of fascia
Culley splint
cuneiform osteotomy
cup
   acetabular
   Arthropor
   Aufranc-Turner acetabular
   Aufranc-Turner hip
   Biomet acetabular
   bipolar acetabular
   bipolar prosthetic
   Buchholz acetabular
   ceramic acetabular
   Charnley acetabular
   Crawford-Adams acetabular
   custom-made acetabular

cup *(cont.)*
   DePuy bipolar
   Hallister heel
   Harris-Galante acetabular
   heel
   Laing concentric hip
   low-profile
   Luck hip
   McKee-Farrar acetabular
   metal-backed acetabular
   migration of acetabular
   Müller-type
   New England Baptist acetabular
   oblong polyethylene acetabular
   Osteonics acetabular
   plastic heel
   press-fit
   retroversion of acetabular
   S-ROM super
   Smith-Petersen
   trial acetabular
   Tuli heel
cup arthroplasty (see *operation*)
curet(te) (noun)
   angled Scoville
   bone
   bowl
   Brun bone
   Cone ring
   curved
   fine
   hex handle
   Kerrison
   long
   McElroy
   oval curved cup
   Scoville
   short
curet, curetted (verb)
curettement, curettings
Curry hip nail
Curtin plantar fibromatosis excision
Curtis PIP joint capsulotomy
Curtis-Fisher knee technique
curvature
   dorsal kyphotic

curvature (cont.)
   humpbacked spinal
   radius of
curve
   flattening of normal lumbar
   lumbar lordotic
   normal lordotic
curvilinear incision
Cushing-Gigli saw guide
Cushing-Hopkins periosteal elevator
cushion
   FB cast
   Sorbothane heel
Cutter cast
cutter
   A-P
   bolt
   bone
   bone plug
   cast
   cookie
   cushion-throat wire
   end
   motorized meniscus
   multiple action
   pin
   side
CVA (costovertebral angle)
cyanoacrylate (Superglue) adhesive
Cybex machine; test
cyst
   aneurysmal bone
   Baker
   bone
   epidermoid
   ganglion
   inclusion
   meniscal
   mucous
   pilonidal
   popliteal
   rheumatoid
   sacral
   synovial
   unicameral bone

# D, d

D-spine (dorsal spine)
Dacron graft
Dacron-impregnated silicone rod
Dakin tubing
DANA shoulder prosthesis
Daniel iliac bone graft
Darrach-McLaughlin shoulder technique
Das Gupta scapulectomy
d'Aubigne femoral reconstruction
Davey-Rorabeck-Fowler decompression technique
Davis muscle-pedicle graft
Dawbarn sign
Day fixation device; pin; staple
DB (Denis Browne) bar
DBM (demineralized bone matrix)
DC (dynamic compression) plate
DCP (dynamic compression plate)
DCS (dorsal column stimulator)
DDT screw
de Andrade-MacNab occipito-cervical arthrodesis
De La Caffiniere trapeziometacarpal prosthesis
de Lange syndrome
de Quervain disease
Dean scissors
Debeyre-Patte-Elmelik rotator cuff technique
debride
debridement
   Ahern trochanteric
   arthroscopic
   Magnuson
debris
   bone
   particulate
debulk, debulking
deburring
decalcification
dechondrification
deciduous

decortication
Decubinex pad/protector
decussation
Dee elbow hinge
deep tendon reflexes (DTR)
deep-shelled acetabulum
defect
  bridging of
  cortical
  developmental
  fusiform
  mapping of the
  nonsubperiosteal cortical
  osseous
  osteochondral
  subcortical
  subperiosteal cortical
  trochlear
defervesce, defervesced, defervescence
deficiency
  Aitken femoral
  factor VIII
  factor IX
deficit, sensory or motor
deformity
  angular
  back-knee
  bifid thumb
  bony
  boutonnière
  bowing
  bunion
  buttonhole
  cavovarus
  checkrein
  clawfoot
  clawhand
  clawtoe
  codfish
  compensatory
  congenital vertical talus foot
  equinovalgus
  eversion-external rotation
  genu valgum
  genu varum
  hatchet-head

deformity *(cont.)*
  internal rotation
  intrinsic minus
  intrinsic plus
  joint
  Kirner
  Madelung
  mallet
  mallet finger
  plantar flexion-inversion
  rotational
  round shoulder
  silver-fork
  Sprengel
  swan-neck finger
  thumb-in-palm
  triphalangeal thumb
  turned-up pulp
  ulnar drift
  valgus
  varus
  Velpeau
  windblown
  windswept
degeneration
  cartilaginous
  wear and tear
degenerative arthritic change
degloving injury
dehiscence, wound
Dehne cast
Dejerine-Sottas disease; syndrome
Delbet splint for heel fracture
Delitala T-nail
deltoid insertion over joint
deltopectoral interval
demarcate, demarcated, demarcation
Demianoff sign
demineralization, bony
demineralized bone matrix (DBM)
DeMuth screw
denatured alcohol
Denham external fixation
Denis Browne talipes hobble splint
Dennyson-Fulford arthrodesis
de novo (over again)

dens (odontoid) x-ray view
densitometry
  bone
  dual-photon
  photon
dental freer
dentinogenesis imperfecta
denude, denuded, denudation
deossification
DePalma modified patellar technique
depression of fragment
DePuy AML Porocoat stem prosthesis
derangement, internal
dermabrader
dermatofibrosarcoma protuberans
dermatomal
dermatome
  Brown
  Reese
  Stryker
dermatomyositis
dermodesis, resection
dermometer
derotate, derotated, derotation
Desault wrist dislocation; bandage
desmalgia
desmectasis
desmitis
desmocytoma
desmodynia
desmoid, cortical
desmoma
desmopathy
desmoplasia
desmoplastic
desmorrhexis
desmosis
desmotomy
Desormaux endoscope
detritus
deviation
  angular
  radial
  rotary
  ulnar
Devic disease

device (see also *apparatus*)
  adjustable aiming
  body-powered prosthetic
  collapsible internal fixation
  compression screw-plate
  coracoclavicular fixation
  coring
  CPM (continuous passive motion)
  driver tunnel locator
  EBI (electronic bone stimulation)
  external fixation
  external skeletal fixation
  fixating
  halo vest
  internal fixation
  leg-holding
  nail-bending
  nail-plate
  rod-mounted targeting
  snap-fit
devitalized tissue
DeWald spinal appliance
Dewar-Barrington clavicular dislocation technique
Dewar-Harris shoulder technique
Dexon suture
dextrorotoscoliosis
dextroscoliosis
Deyerle II pin; plate
DF80 (Wilson-Burstein) hip internal prosthesis
diacondylar fracture
diadochokinesia, diadochokinesis
diagnostic arthroscopy and debridement
dial-lock brace
Diamond nail
Diamond-Gould syndactyly operation
diapering, triple
diaphysectomy
diaphysis, diaphyses, diaphyseal
diaplasis
diarthrosis
Dias-Giegerich fracture technique
diastasis, diastatic
diastematomyelia

diastrophic dwarfism
diathermy
　microwave (MWD)
　shortwave (SWD)
Dickhaut-DeLee classification of discoid meniscus
Dickinson calcaneal bursitis technique
Dickinson-Coutts-Woodward-Handler osteotomy
Dickson transplant technique
diet
　low purine
　tea-and-toast
digit
　accessory
　supernumerary
digital color (color of digit)
digital opposers
digitorum
digitus
dilator, Eder-Puestow metal olive
Dimon-Hughston fracture fixation
dimple the bone
Dingman mouth gag
DIP (distal interphalangeal) joint
DiPalma shoe lift
diphasic
diplegia
diploscope
director, grooved
disability, permanent
disarticulate, disarticulation
disarticulation
　Batch-Spittler-McFaddin knee
　Boyd hip
　elbow
　wrist
disc (see *disk*)
discectomy (see *diskectomy*)
discogenic
discogram (also *diskogram*)
discography (see *diskography*)
discoid lateral meniscus
discrepancy, leg length
discrete blood supply to a bone graft
discrimination, two-point

discus, disci
disease (also *disorder*)
　Albers-Schönberg
　Apert
　Atton
　Blount
　Brodie
　Caffey
　caisson worker's
　Calve-Perthes
　Charcot joint
　Charcot-Marie-Tooth
　Christmas hemophiliac
　congenital disorder (skeletal hypoplasia)
　connective tissue
　de Quervain
　degenerative disk
　degenerative disorder (osteoarthritis)
　degenerative joint (DJD)
　Dejerine-Sottas
　developmental disorder (scoliosis)
　Devic
　diver's
　Duchenne
　Duplay
　end-organ
　Engelmann
　Erb-Goldflam
　Erb-Landouzy
　Erdheim-Chester
　Erhenfeld
　fibromuscular
　Forestier
　Freiberg
　Friedreich
　Garre
　Gaucher
　Gilbert
　Hand-Schüller-Christian
　histiocytosis X group
　Hurler
　Jaffe
　Kienböck
　Kimura
　Köhler

disease | 38 | dislocation

disease *(cont.)*
　König
　Kugelberg-Welander
　Kümmell
　Landouzy-Dejerine
　Legg-Calve-Perthes
　Legg-Perthes
　Letterer-Siwe
　lipid storage
　Lou Gehrig
　lower motor neuron
　Lyme
　Marie-Bamberger
　Marie-Charcot-Tooth
　Marie-Strümpell
　milk-alkali
　Milroy
　Morquio
　neoplastic disorder
　neurologic
　Niemann-Pick
　Ollier
　Oppenheim
　Osgood-Schlatter
　Paget
　Panner
　Pellegrini-Stieda
　Perthes
　Peyronie
　Scheuermann
　Sever
　Sinding-Larsen-Johansson
　Still
　Sudeck
　Thiemann
　Thomsen
　traumatic disorder (fracture)
　upper motor neuron
　von Recklinghausen
　Voorhoeve
　Werdnig-Hoffman
　DISH (diffuse idiopathic sclerosing hyperostosis, or diffuse idiopathic skeletal hyperostosis)
　DISI (dorsal intercalary segment instability)

disjointing
disk (also *disc)*
　bulging
　crescent-shaped
　fibrocartilaginous
　herniated cervical
　intervertebral
　massive herniated
　midline herniation of
　protruding
　ruptured
　sequestered
　slipped
Diskard head halter
diskectomy (also *discectomy)*
　cervical
　Cloward fusion
　microlumbar
　Williams
diskitis
diskogram
diskography, cervical (also *discography)*
disk protrusion
dislocated knee, or patella
dislocation
　anterior hip
　anterior-inferior
　Bankart shoulder
　Bell-Dally cervical
　Bennett
　boutonnière hand
　bursting
　carpometacarpal
　central
　Chopart ankle
　closed
　complete
　compound
　congenital, of the hip (CDH)
　consecutive
　Desault wrist
　divergent elbow
　frank
　gamekeeper's
　habitual
　Hill-Sach shoulder

dislocation *(cont.)*
  incomplete
  isolated
  Kienböck
  knee
  Lisfranc
  lunate
  luxatio erecta shoulder
  metacarpophalangeal
  milkmaid's elbow
  Monteggia
  Nélaton ankle
  open
  Otto pelvis
  partial
  pathologic
  perilunate carpal
  posterior hip
  primitive
  recurrent
  simple
  Smith
  subastragalar
  subcoracoid shoulder
  subglenoid shoulder
  talar
  tarsal
  tarsometatarsal
  transscaphoid perilunate
  traumatic
  triquetrolunate
  volar semilunar wrist
disorder (see *disease*)
displacement, Ellis Jones peroneal
  tendon
disruption
  joint
  ligamentous
dissection
  blunt
  bone
  extracapsular
  field of
  sharp
  subperiosteal

dissector
  bunion
  grooved
  Penfield
disseminated-type pigmented villonodular synovitis
dissipate
distal third of shaft
distalward
disto-occlusal
distract, distracting, distraction
distraction of fracture
distractor
  femoral
  Santa Casa
divot
DJD (degenerative joint disease)
DMI orthopedic bed
DOA (diagnostic and operative
  arthroscopy)
dog-ear
dolichostenomelia
Doll trochanteric reattachment
  technique
dome
  shoulder
  talar
  weightbearing acetabular
Don Joy knee brace
Donati suture
donor team
Dooley nail
Doppler ultrasound segmental blood
  pressure testing
Dorrance hand prosthesis
dorsal spine (D1 to D12)
dorsalis pedis pulse
dorsalward
dorsiflexion, dorsiflexors
dorsolateral and medial capsulotomy
dorsomedial incision
dorsoplantar view
dorsoradial
dorsum
Dow Corning Wright prosthesis
dowel, doweled, doweling

dowel spinal fusion
doweling spondylolisthesis technique
Down syndrome
Downey hemilaminectomy retractor
drain
  Hemovac
  Jackson-Pratt
  Nélaton rubber tube
  Penrose
  rubber
  Silastic
drape
  fenestrated
  Loban adhesive
  3M skin
draped out
Drennan metaphyseal-epiphyseal angle
dressing (see also *bandage*)
  ABD
  ACU-derm wound
  Adaptic
  Aeroplast
  Aquaphor
  Betadine
  Bioclusive transparent
  bulky
  Bunnell
  Coban
  collodion
  compression, compressive
  Conform
  cotton
  Coverlet adhesive surgical
  Cover-Roll adhesive gauze
  dry
  Duoderm
  Elastikon
  Elastomull
  Elastoplast
  Esmarch
  figure-of-8
  Flexinet
  fluff
  Fuller shield
  Furacin gauze
  gauze

dressing *(cont.)*
  Glasscock ear
  iodoform gauze
  Jones
  Kerlix
  Kling adhesive
  Koch-Mason
  Lyofoam
  Microfoam
  nonadherent gauze
  Nu-gauze
  O'Donoghue
  occlusive
  Op-Site
  palm-to-axilla
  patch
  pledget
  pressure
  rigid
  Robert Jones
  Shanz
  silk mesh gauze
  Sof-Wick
  soft bulky
  stent
  sterile
  Tegaderm
  Telfa gauze
  toe-to-groin modified Jones
  Velpeau
  Vigilon
  Webril
  wet-to-dry
  wide-mesh petroleum gauze
  Xeroform gauze
Dreyer formula
Drez modification of Eriksson technique
Driessen hinged plate
drill
  Adson
  air-powered cutting
  Anspach power
  battery-driven hand
  biflanged
  bone

drill *(cont.)*
  Bosworth
  Bunnell hand
  cannulated
  cement eater
  centering
  cervical
  Charnley centering
  Cherry-Austin
  chuck
  Cloward
  Codman
  Collison
  cortical
  Crutchfield
  Cushing
  D'Errico perforator
  dental
  Gray
  Hall air
  hand
  hand-operated
  high-speed twist
  Mathews
  Osteone air
  pilot
  right-angle dental
  Shea
  Zimmer hand
drill bit, cannulated
drill point
  cannulated
  carbon steel
drive, worm
driver
  blade plate
  bullet
  Flatt
  Harrington hook
  Jewett
  Küntscher
  Massie
  nail
  prosthesis
  staple
  supine position

driver-bender-extractor, Rush
driver-extractor
  Hansen-Street
  Ken
  McReynolds
  Sage
  Schneider
  Zimmer
drop foot
Drummond wire technique
Dryspell cast cover
DTR (deep tendon reflex)
dual-lock hip prosthesis
dual-photon densitometry test for osteoporosis
Duchenne muscular atrophy; dystrophy
Dugas test
Duncan prone rectus test
Dunlop traction
Dunlop-Shands view
Dunn-Brittain foot stabilization technique
Dunn-Hess trochanteric osteotomy
Duo-Driv screw
Duoderm dressing
Duopress guide; plate
Dupaco knee control; prosthesis
Duplay disease
Dupuytren contracture release
Duran-Houser wrist splint
Durham flatfoot
duToit-Roux staple capsulorrhaphy
Duverney's fracture
DuVries deltoid ligament reconstruction technique
DuVries-Mann bunionectomy
dwarfism
  achondroplastic
  diastrophic
Dwyer cable for correction of scoliosis
Dwyer-Wickham electrical stimulation
Dycal base
Dyck-Lambert classification
Dyna knee splint
Dynagrip handle of blade
dynamometer, Jamar

Dynaplex knee prosthesis
Dyonics Golden Retriever magnet
Dyonics cannula; shaver
dysautonomia
dysbasia, dysbaric
dyschondroplasia
dyscrasia, dyscratic
dysdiadochokinesia
dysesthesia
dysfunction
dysgenesis
  alar
  epiphyseal
dyskinesia, dyskinetic
dysmetria
dysostosis, cleidocranial
dysplasia
  congenital hip
  diaphyseal
  epiarticular osteochondromatous
  fibrous
  monostotic fibrous
  multiple epiphyseal
  oculoauriculovertebral
  polyostotic fibrous
  progressive diaphyseal
  spondyloepiphyseal
dystaxia
dystonia
dystrophy
  Becker muscular
  Duchenne muscular
  facioscapulohumeral muscular
  Fröhlich adiposogenital
  juvenile muscular
  muscular
  myotonic muscular
  pseudohypertrophic muscular
  reflex sympathetic

# E, e

Eagle arthroscope
EAST (external rotation, abduction stress test)
East-West retractor
Eaton-Littler technique
Eaton-Malerich fracture-dislocation technique
Eberle contracture release technique
EBI (electronic bone stimulation)
eburnated, eburnation
ecchondroma
ecchondrotome
ecchymosis
Ecker-Lotke-Glazer tendon reconstruction technique
ECRB (extensor carpi radialis brevis)
ECRL (extensor carpi radialis longus)
ECU (extensor carpi ulnaris)
EDC (extensor digitorum communis)
edema
  dependent
  intracompartmental
  mushy
  nonpitting
  pitting
  pretibial
edematous
Eden-Hybbinette arthroplasty
Eden-Lange procedure
Eder-Puestow metal olive dilator
EDF scoliosis cast
EDL (extensor digitorum longus)
EDQ (extensor digiti quinti)
Edward procedure
effect
  doorstopper
  halo (x-ray)
  lag
effusion, bloody
Eftekhar broken femoral stem technique
Egawa sign
Eggers plate; screw; splint

Eggers tendon transfer technique
EHL (extensor hallucis longus) tendon
Ehlers-Danlos syndrome
Eicher femoral prosthesis
EIP (extensor indicis proprius)
elasticity, modulus of
Elastikon elastic tape for pressure dressings
elastofibroma dorsi
Elastomull elastic gauze bandage
Elastoplast bandage; dressing
elbow
    baseball pitcher's
    boxer's
    floating
    javelin thrower's
    Little Leaguer's
    milkmaid's
    reverse tennis
    tennis
elbow prosthesis (see *prosthesis*)
elective surgery
electrocautery apparatus
electrocoagulated
electrode, surface
electrodesiccated bleeding points
electromyogram, electromyography (EMG)
electromyographic study
electrostimulation (pulsing current) for nonunion of fracture
elevate on pillows
elevation of extremity
elevator
    Adson periosteal
    Aufranc periosteal
    Bennett
    Bethune periosteal
    Blair
    Bowen periosteal
    Bristow periosteal
    Brophy periosteal
    Cameron-Haight periosteal
    Carroll-Legg periosteal
    Chandler
    Cheyne periosteal

elevator *(cont.)*
    chisel-edge
    Cloward periosteal
    Cobb
    Cobb periosteal
    Coryllos-Doyen periosteal
    curved periosteal
    Cushing-Hopkins periosteal
    Darrach
    Freer
    Gardner
    Harrington spinal
    Hoen
    J-periosteal
    joker periosteal
    Key
    Key periosteal
    Langenbeck periosteal
    Locke
    nasal
    Penfield
    periosteal
    Sheffield hand
    straight periosteal
    Tegtmeier
    von Langenbeck periosteal
elevator-dissector, Freer
Elizabethtown method osteotomy
Elliott femoral condyle blade plate
ellipsoid joint
elliptical
Ellis Jones peroneal tendon technique
Ellis technique for Barton fracture
Ellison lateral knee reconstruction
Elmslie-Trillat patellar procedure
elongation derotation flexion
ELP broach; femoral prosthesis
Ely test
embarrassment, circulatory
embolus, embolism
    air
    fat
emergency closed manipulative measure
EMG (electromyogram; electromyography)

eminence
  hypothenar
  medial
  thenar
Emmon osteotomy
empirical
empyema
emulsified
en bloc
en face
encerclage
enchondral ossification
enchondroma
enchondromatosis
encroachment, bony
end point
Ender femoral fracture technique
endochondral ossification
endoprosthesis (see *prosthesis*)
endoscope, Desormaux
endosteal surface
endotracheal intubation
Engel plaster saw
Engel-May nail
Engelmann disease
Englehardt femoral prosthesis
Englemann splint
Enneking staging of malignant soft tissue tumor
entrapment, popliteal
enucleate, enucleation
eosinophilic granuloma
EPB (extensor pollicis brevis)
ependymoma
epicondylar fracture
epicondyle, epicondylitis
  lateral
  medial
epidermoid cyst
epidurography
epimysium
epineural covering
epineurial neurorrhaphy
epineurium, epineurial
epineurolysis, volar
epineurosis

epiphyseal hyperplasia
epiphysealis
epiphysiodesis
  Blount
  bone peg
  White
epiphysis, epiphyses
  capital femoral
  capitular
  stippled
  tibial
epiphysitis
epithelioid sarcoma
epitrochlea, epitrochlear
EPL (extensor pollicis longus)
eponychium
Eppright dial osteotomy
equinocavovarus
equinovalgus, spastic
equinovarus, talipes
equinus, talipes
Erb-Duchenne palsy
Erb-Goldflam disease
Erb-Landouzy disease
Erdheim-Chester disease
ERE (external rotation in extension)
erector spinae
ERF (external rotation in flexion)
ergometer
Erhenfeld disease
Erich splint
Erichsen sign
Erickson-Leider-Brown technique
Eriksson ligament technique
erosion of articular surface
erysipelas
erythema of joint
erythrocyte sedimentation rate (ESR)
eschar, escharotic
Esmarch bandage; tourniquet
ESR (erythrocyte sedimentation rate)
Essex-Lopresti axial fixation technique
esthesia
estimated blood loss (EBL)
Ethibond suture

Ethilon suture
Evans ankle reconstruction technique
eventration
eversion, ankle
everted, eversion
evertors
Ewald-Walker kinematic knee
  arthroplasty
EWHO (elbow-wrist-hand orthosis)
Ewing sarcoma; tumor
exacerbated, exacerbation
exarticulation
excision of intervertebral disk
excision of osteochondroma
excision (see *operation*)
excoriation
excrescence, bony
excursion, range of
Exer-Cor exerciser
exerciser
  Exer-Cor
  Nelson finger
exercises
  active range of motion
  active assisted range of motion
  ankle pump
  Calleja
  Codman
  external rotation
  graded
  hamstring-setting
  hip abductor strengthening
  internal rotation
  inversion-eversion
  isometric
  knee pump
  muscle-setting
  passive range of motion
  pendulum
  progressive resistive
  pulley
  quad-set (quadriceps-setting)
  quad strengthening
  range of motion
  Regen flexion
  resistive

exercises *(cont.)*
  straight leg raising
  supported extension
  Williams flexion
Exeter hip prosthesis
exogenous
exostectomy
exostoses, hereditary multiple
exostosis
  epiphyseal
  hypertrophic
  turret
expander, acetabular
exploration and debridement
exploration and revision
exsanguinate, exsanguinated
exsanguination
exstrophy
extender, nail
extension
  headrest
  Hittenberger halo
  toe plate
extensor carpi radialis brevis (ECRB)
extensor carpi radialis longus (ECRL)
extensor digitorum communis (EDC)
extensor digitorum longus (EDL)
extensor hallucis longus (EHL) tendon
extensor indicis proprius musculus
extensors, wrist
external fixation (see *apparatus*)
external rotation in extension (ERE)
external rotation in flexion (ERF)
extirpation
extra-articular resection
extracapsular dissection
extractor
  Austin Moore
  bone
  Cherry
  cloverleaf pin
  corkscrew femoral head
  FIN
  femoral head
  Küntscher
  Massie

extractor *(cont.)*
   Moore prosthesis
   Nicoll
   staple
extractor-driver, Schneider
extractor-impactor, Fox
extramedullary plasmacytoma
extravasation
extremity, extremities
extrusion, disk
exude, exudate
Eyler flexorplasty

# F, f

fabella
fabellofibular complex
fabere (flexion, abduction, external rotation, extension) sign, test
facet tropism
facetectomy, O'Donoghue
facies
facioscapulohumeral muscular dystrophy
factor VIII deficiency
factor IX deficiency
factor, RA (rheumatoid arthritis)
fadir (flexion, adduction, internal rotation) sign, test
Fahey-Compere pin
failure of conservative management
Fairbanks-Sever procedure
Fajersztajn crossed sciatic sign
Fanconi syndrome
Farmer operation
Fas-Trac strips
fascia
   antebrachial
   clavipectoral
   crural
   deltoid

fascia *(cont.)*
   investing
   lumbar
   medial geniculate
   palmar
   plantar
   quadratus femoris
fascia lata (*but* tensor fasciae latae)
fascial arthroplasty
fasciaplasty (also *fascioplasty*)
fasciatome
fascicle, fascicular
fasciculus, fasciculi
fasciectomy, partial
fasciitis
   necrotizing
   nodular
fasciodesis
fasciogram
fasciorrhaphy
fasciotomy, subcutaneous
fat, subcutaneous
fatigue strength
fat pad, heel
FB cast cushion
FCR (flexor carpi radialis)
FCU (flexor carpi ulnaris)
FDL (flexor digitorum longus)
FDP (flexor digitorum profundus)
FDQB (flexor digiti quinti brevis)
FDS (flexor digitorum sublimis)
felon infection
felt
   orthopedic
   rolled
femoral prosthesis (see *prosthesis*)
femur, femora, femoral
fenestrated drape
Fenton bolt
Ferciot-Thomson excision
Ferguson-Thompson-King two-stage osteotomy
Ferkel torticollis technique
Fernandez osteotomy
Ferris-Smith rongeur
festinating gait

Fett prosthesis
FFC (fixed flexion contracture)
fiber(s)
    annular
    collagen
    Sharpey
    tendinous
fiberoptic light source
fibers, Sharpey
fibrillation
fibroblast
fibrocartilaginous plate
fibroma molle
fibroma molluscum
fibroma
    aponeurotic
    chondromyxoid
    nonossifying
    osteogenic
    periosteal
fibromatosis
    fascial
    infantile dermal
    irradiation
fibromatosis colli
fibromuscular disease
fibromyositis
fibro-osseous tunnel
fibrosarcoma
fibrositis, periarticular
fibrous dysplasia ossificans progressiva
fibrous union
fibroxanthoma
fibular ostectomy
Ficat operation
field of dissection
field
    bloodless
    pulsating electromagnetic (PEMF)
Fielding-Magliato classification of subtrochanteric fracture
figure 4 position
file, bone
file, filed
filiform
Fillauer night splint

filler, shoe
film, scout
filter, Greenfield
finger(s)
    lumbrical plus
    football
    index
    little
    long
    mallet
    middle
    pulp of
    ring
    spider
    trigger
finger intrinsics
finger-trap suspension
fingerbreadth(s)
fingernail, base of
fingertrap, Chinese
Finkelstein sign (test) for synovitis
FIN pin guide
Fischer ring
Fish cuneiform osteotomy technique
Fisher guide; rasp
fisticuffs
Fitron
fitting
    immediate postsurgical (IPSF)
    prosthetic
    Velcro
fix, fixation *(not* fixate)
fixation (see *operation*)
    bolt
    bone-ingrowth
    circumferential wire loop
    Cole tendon
    dynamic
    external
    four-bar external
    greenstick
    internal
    monofilament wire
    nail
    pin
    screw-and-plate

fixation *(cont.)*
  screw-and-wire
  static
  tension band
  wire
fixation device (see *apparatus; device)*
fixator
  Ace-Colles external
  Ace-Fischer external
  Claiborne external
  Hoffman external
  Orthofix
flaccid, flaccidity
Flanagan-Burem apposing hemicylindric graft
flange
flap congestion
flap graft, Kutler V-Y
flap
  abdominal
  advancement
  Atasoy triangular advancement
  axial pattern
  bipedicle
  cross-finger
  hemipulp
  horseshoe-shaped
  iliofemoral pedicle
  musculocutaneous free flap
  musculotendinous
  pulp
  radial-based
  remote pedicle
  skin
  thenar
  transposition
  wraparound
flare of the condyle
flatfoot
  Durham procedure for
  rockerbottom
Flatt finger/thumb prosthesis
flattening of normal lumbar curve
Fleck sign
flex against gravity
flex, flexed, flexion

flex, forward
Flex-Foam bandage
Flex-Master bandage
flexion and extension
flexion-rotation-compression maneuvers
flexion
  dorsiflexion
  elongation-derotation
  plantar
flexor carpi ulnaris
flexor pollicis longus
flexor wad of five
flexorplasty
  Bunnell modification of Steindler
  Eyler
  Steindler
flexors and extensors
flocculent foci of calcification
floor of the acetabulum
Florida cervical brace
Flotan thumb
fluid, synovial
fluorescein perfusion monitoring
fluoroscopy
  portable C-arm image intensifier
  two-plane
flush, peroxide
flutes of cannulated screw
Flynn technique
foot
  Charcot
  clawfoot
  drop
  flatfoot
  march
  Morton
  rockerbottom
  SACH (solid-ankle, cushioned heel)
  sole of
  splay
  Syme prosthetic
  tabetic
foot-ankle assembly
footdrop
foot orthosis (see *orthosis)*

foot piece
  Bunker
  traction
footplate, metal
foot pound
foot prosthesis (see *prosthesis*)
footwear
forage procedure
foramen of Froesch
foramen, foramina, foraminal
foraminotomy
Forbes modification of Phemister graft
  technique
force
  Newton
  torque
forceps
  Acufex curved basket
  Acufex rotary biting basket
  Allis
  arthroscopy basket
  arthroscopy grasping
  Asch
  Backhaus towel
  basket
  bipolar
  Boies
  bone-biting
  bone-breaking
  bone-cutting
  bone-grasping
  bone-holding
  bone-splitting
  Hoen
  jeweler's
  Kelly
  Kern bone-holding
  Lane self-retaining bone-holding
  plain tissue
  ring
  Rowe disimpaction
  Russian
  Stille-Liston bone-cutting
  three-edge cutting
  toothed tissue
  vascular

forces, tension
forearm lift-assist on prosthesis
forefoot splaying
Forestier disease
fork strap prosthetic support
formation
  bunion
  callus
  osteophyte
  new bone
  rouleaux
  forme fruste
formula, Dreyer
Forrester splint
Forrester-Brown head halter
Forte harness
fossa ovalis
Foster bed; frame; splint
four-point walker
four-poster cervical orthosis
Fournier test
fovea
Fowler maneuver; procedure
Fowles dislocation technique
Fox extractor-impactor; splint
Fox-Blazina procedure
FPB (flexor pollicis brevis)
FPL (flexor pollicis longus)
Frac-Sur splint
Fractura Flex cast
fracture
  agenetic
  anatomic
  angulated
  ankle mortise
  apophyseal
  articular
  Atkin epiphyseal
  atrophic
  avulsion
  Barton
  basal neck
  baseball finger
  basilar femoral neck
  bending
  Bennett

[handwritten: ?Schatzker V (sp'? peRBJ)]

fracture 50 fracture

fracture *(cont.)*
  bicondylar
  bimalleolar ankle
  blow-out
  boot-top
  both-bone
  boxer's
  bucket-handle
  bunk bed
  bursting
  butterfly
  buttonhole
  cartwheel
  cementum
  cervicotrochanteric
  Chance
  chauffeur [handwritten: Chopart]
  chip
  chisel
  clay shoveler's
  cleavage
  closed
  closed break
  Colles'
  comminuted
  complete
  complex
  complicated
  composite
  compound
  compression
  condylar
  congenital
  contrecoup
  cortical
  Cotton ankle
  dashboard
  depressed
  diacondylar
  diastatic
  dislocation, transscaphoid
  displaced
  dogleg
  dome
  double

fracture *(cont.)*
  Dupuytren
  Duverney
  dyscrasic
  epicondylar
  epiphyseal slip
  Essex-Lopresti calcaneal
  extracapsular
  fatigue
  femoral neck
  fissure
  Frykman radial
  Galeazzi
  Garden femoral neck
  Gosselin
  greenstick
  hairline
  hamate tail
  hangman's
  hemicondylar
  hickory-stick
  hockey-stick
  horizontal
  humeral head-splitting
  impacted
  incomplete
  inflammatory
  infraction
  interperiosteal
  intertrochanteric
  intra-articular
  intracapsular
  irreducible
  Jefferson
  Jones
  Kocher
  Le Fort
  lead pipe
  linear
  Lisfranc
  long bone
  longitudinal
  loose
  Maisonneuve fibular
  Malgaigne pelvic

Gardener IV (?fracture)

fracture (cont.)
 mallet
 malunited
 march
 midshaft
 monomalleolar ankle
 Monteggia
 Montercaux
 Moore
 multangular ridge
 navicular
 naviculocapitate
 neoplastic
 neurogenic
 neuropathic
 nightstick
 nondisplaced
 oblique
 occult
 open
 open-break
 osteochondral
 Pais
 paratrooper
 parry
 patellar
 pathologic
 Pauwels
 pedicle
 periarticular
 Piedmont
 pillion
 pillow
 ping-pong
 pond
 posterior element
 Pott ankle
 pyramidal
 Quervain
 radial head
 reverse Barton
 reverse Colles
 ring
 Rolando
 Salter I-VI
 Salter-Harris

fracture (cont.)
 secondary
 segmental
 Segond
 SER-IV
 shaft
 Shepherd
 sideswipe elbow
 silver-fork
 simple
 skier's
 Skillern
 Smith
 spiral
 splintered
 spontaneous
 sprain
 sprinter's
 stairstep
 stellate
 Stieda
 stress
 subcapital
 subperiosteal
 subtrochanteric
 supracondylar
 surgical neck
 T
 T condylar
 teardrop
 through-and-through
 tibial plafond
 tibial plateau
 Tillaux
 torsion
 torus
 transcapitate
 transcervical femoral
 transcondylar
 transhamate
 transcaphoid
 transtriquetral
 trimalleolar ankle
 triplane
 triquetral
 trophic

fracture *(cont.)*
   tuft
   undisplaced
   unstable
   vertebra plana
   vertebral wedge compression
   vertical shear
   wagon wheel
   Wagstaffe
   wedge
   willow
   Y
   Y-T
fracture by contrecoup
fracture classification (see *classification*)
fracture-dislocation (see *fracture*)
fracture en coin
fracture en rave
fracture frame (see *frame*)
fracture nonunion
   elephant-foot
   horse-hoof
   oligotrophic
   torsion wedge
fracture table (see *table*)
fragilitas ossium congenita
fragment(s)
   alignment of fracture
   articular
   bony
   butterfly fracture
   chondral
   cortical
   disk
   free
   free-floating cartilaginous
   loose
   osteochondral
frame
   Ace-Colles fracture
   Ace-Fischer fracture
   Ace-Fischer ring
   Alexian Brothers overhead
   Balkan fracture
   Böhler fracture

frame *(cont.)*
   Böhler reducing
   Böhler-Braun
   Bradford fracture
   Braun
   Brooker
   Charest head
   CircOlectric
   claw-type basic
   Cole fracture
   Cole hyperextension
   Crawford head
   DePuy rainbow
   DePuy reducing
   Foster turning
   Goldthwait
   Granberry
   Hastings
   Herzmark
   Hibbs
   Hoffman-Vidal double
   Jones abduction
   laminectomy
   Pittsburgh pelvic
   scoliosis operating
   Slätis pelvic fracture
   spine
   Stryker fracture
   Stryker turning
   Taylor spinal
   Thomas
   Thompson
   vasocillator
   Wagner
   Whitman
   Wilson
   Wingfield
   Zimmer laminectomy
Fränkel white line; sign
fray, frayed, fraying
Frazier suction tip
free flap transfer
free revascularized autogroft
Freeman-Samuelson prosthesis
Freeman-Swanson knee prosthesis
Freer elevator-dissector

freeze-drying (lyophilization)
Freiberg meniscectomy knife
Frejka cast; jacket; pillow
fremitus
French fracture technique
French scale for sizing catheters, sounds, etc.
frenectomy
frenulum
freshen the surface
friable
Fried-Hendel tendon technique
Friedman brace; support
Friedreich ataxia; disease; sign
fringe, synovial
Fröhlich adiposogenital dystrophy
Froimson procedure
Froment paper sign
frond, synovial
F.R. Thompson femoral prosthesis
Fruehevald splint
Frykman classification of fracture
FTSG (full-thickness skin graft)
fulgurate, fulgurated
full-thickness skin graft (FTSG)
fulminate
funiculus
Funsten splint
Furnas-Haq-Somers technique
fuse, fused, fusion
fusiform
fusion (see also *operation*)
    ankle
    anterior spinal
    atlanto-occipital
    calcaneotibial
    cervical interbody
    dowel spinal
    extra-articular hip
    intra-articular knee
    posterior spinal
    posterior cervical
    posterolateral
    symmetric vertebral
    tibiotalar fusion
    two-stage

fusion of two or more vertebral segments
fx (fracture)

# G, g

G suit
Gaenslen split heel incision
Gage sign
Gagnon splint
gait
    antalgic
    apraxic
    calcaneous
    cogwheel
    drop foot
    dystrophic
    equine
    festinating
    four-point
    free-swinging knee
    glue-footed
    gluteal
    heel
    heel-and-toe
    hemiplegic
    hysterical
    listing
    Oppenheim
    propulsion
    scissor
    shuffling
    spastic
    stable
    stance phase of
    steppage
    swing-through
    swing-to
    tabetic
    three-point
    Trendelenburg

*Handwritten at top:* Genutrain brace (5'/ per Tracey Hughston)

| gait | 54 | glabella |

*Handwritten:* Galvanic unit per T. Carpenter

gait *(cont.)*
   two-point
   waddling
gait and station
gait training
Gaiter cast
Galant sign
Galeazzi patellar operation
Gallannaugh plate
Gallie atlantoaxial fusion technique
Gallo traction
gammopathy, monoclonal
ganglion, Acrel
ganglioneuroma
gangrene, gas
Gant osteotomy
Garceau tendon technique
Garceau cheilectomy
Garceau-Brahms arthrodesis
Garden femoral neck fracture
Gardner chair; elevator
Gardner-Wells tong traction
Garre, sclerosing osteomyelitis of
Gartland classification of supra-
   condylar fracture
gastrocnemius, lateral head
Gatch bed
gatched bed
Gatellier-Chastang ankle approach
Gaucher disease
gauge
   acetabular
   bone screw ruler
   Cobb
   depth
   screw depth
   socket
gauntlet, Jobst
gauze (see *dressing*)
Gaynor-Hart x-ray position of carpal
   tunnel
Geckler screw
Geiger counter
gelatin foam, thrombin-soaked
gelatinous
Gelfoam stamps

Gelfoam, thrombin-soaked
Gelocast
Gelpi retractor
gemellus (pl. gemelli) muscle
geniculum, genicular, geniculate
genu recurvatum
genu valgum (knock-knee) deformity
genu varum (bowleg) deformity
Geomedic total knee prosthesis
Geometric total knee prosthesis
Georgiade visor halo fixation
   apparatus
Gerard prosthesis
Gerdy tubercle in knee; ligament
germinal matrix
Gerota capsule
Gerster traction bar
Getty decompression technique
Ghon-Sachs complex
Ghormley arthrodesis
Giannestras modification of Lapidus
   technique
gibbous
Gibney bandage
Gibson approach; bandage; splint
Gibson-Piggott osteotomy
Gigli saw guide
Gilbert-Tamai-Weiland technique
Giliberty bipolar femoral head
Gill sliding graft technique
Gill-Manning-White spondylolisthesis
   technique
Gill-Stein arthrodesis
Gillies-Millard cocked-hat technique
Gillis suture
Gilmer splint
girdle
   limb
   pelvic
   shoulder
Girdlestone resection arthroplasty
Girdlestone-Taylor procedure
Gissane spike
give-way phenomena
giving way of knee
glabella

*Handwritten at bottom:* Gardener IV position.

gland, haversian
Glasgow screw
Glass-Bessen transfixion screw
glenohumeral joint subluxation
glenoid component, keel of
glenoplasty
glioma
Glisson sling
globose
glue, skin
gluteal bonnet
gluteal lurch
gluteus maximus muscle
gluteus maximus tensing test
gluteus medius muscle
gluteus minimus muscle
Glynn-Neibauer technique
gold salts
Goldenhar syndrome
Goldner-Clippinger technique
Goldstein spinal fusion technique
Goldthwait-Hauser procedure
goniometer
Gooch splint
Goodman orthopedic bed
Gordon splint
Gordon-Broström technique
Gordon-Taylor technique
Gore bit
Gore-Tex knee prosthesis; graft; suture
Gore-Tex nonabsorbable surgical suture
Gosselin fracture
Gouffon pin fixation
gouge
    Abbott
    Alexander
    Andrews
    Army bone
    arthroplasty
    Aufranc
    Bishop
    bone
    Campbell
    Cobb
    curved
    gooseneck

gouge *(cont.)*
    Hibbs
    Meyerding
    oscillating
    Smith-Petersen curved; straight
    straight
    swan-neck
gout, tophaceous
Gower sign
grabber, disk
graft
    advancement flap
    Albee bone
    allogenic bone
    anterior sliding tibial
    autogenous bone
    Banks bone
    bone
    bone peg
    Bonfiglio
    Boyd dual onlay bone
    bridge
    Calcitite
    Campbell onlay
    cancellous and cortical bone
    cancellous chip bone
    carbon fiber
    cartilage
    chip
    clothespin spinal fusion
    Codivilla bone
    composite
    cortical
    cortical strut
    corticocancellous bone
    Dacron
    Daniel iliac bone
    Davis muscle-pedicle
    demineralized bone
    devitalized bone
    diamond inlay
    dual onlay bone
    extra-articular
    fillet local flap
    Flanagan-Burem apposing
        hemicylindric

graft *(cont.)*
  free
  free fat
  free skin
  freeze-dried
  full-thickness skin
  Gillies bone
  Gore-Tex vascular
  Haldeman bone
  Harris superior acetabular
  hemicylindrical bone
  Henderson onlay bone
  Henry bone
  heterogeneous (heterogenous)
  Hey-Groves-Kirk bone
  Hoaglund bone
  homogeneous (homogenous)
  homologous
  Huntington bone
  iliac bone
  iliac crest
  Inclan bone
  inlay bone
  intercalary
  interfascicular nerve
  intramedullary
  Judet
  keystone
  Kutler V-Y flap
  Langenskiöld bone
  Lee bone
  lyophilized bone
  Massie sliding
  matchstick
  McFarland bone
  McMaster bone
  medullary bone
  nerve
  neurovascular island
  Nicoll cancellous bone; insert
  nontubed closed distant flap
  nontubed open distant flap
  Ollier thick split free
  onlay cancellous iliac
  osteoarticular
  osteochondral

graft *(cont.)*
  osteoperiosteal
  Overton dowel
  Papineau
  pedicle
  Phemister onlay bone
  porous polyethylene
  postage stamp
  Reverdin epidermal free
  Russe bone
  Ryerson bone
  sandwiched iliac bone
  segmental
  single onlay cortical bone
  skin
  sliding inlay
  Soto-Hall bone
  split-thickness skin
  strut
  Thiersch medium split free
  Thiersch thin split free
  Thomas extrapolated bar
  tube flap
  Wilson bone
  Wolf full-thickness free
  Wolfe-Kawamoto bone
  wraparound flap bone
  Z-plasty local flap
grafting, Papineau
Graham nerve hook
Granberry frame; splint; traction
Grantham classification of femur
  fracture
granuloma
  eosinophilic
  swimming pool
graph, Moseley straight line
graspers, pituitary
grasping power
grate, grating
gravity, flex against
Gray drill
gray matter
Grayson ligament in hand
great toe push-off
Green procedure; transfer

Green-Anderson growth table
Green-Banks technique
Greenfield classification of
  spinocerebellar ataxia
Greenfield filter; osteotomy
Greulich and Pyle, bone age
Grice-Green arthrodesis
grind, grinding
grinder, DePuy calcar
grip tester, Jamar
grip, key
Gristina-Webb total shoulder
  arthroplasty
Gritti-Stokes knee prosthesis
grommet
groove
  annular
  bicipital
  deltopectoral
  femoral
  parasagittal
  patellar
  patellofemoral
  spiral
  trochlear
Grosse-Kempf interlocking medullary
  nailing
Groves-Goldner technique
growth plate, cartilaginous
GSB (Gschwind-Scheier-Bahler) elbow
  prosthesis
guarding, muscle
Guepar hinged knee prosthesis
guide
  acetabular
  ACL drill
  Acufex tibial
  Adson saw
  alignment
  Bailey-Gigli saw
  ball-tipped Küntscher
  Blair saw
  calibrated pin
  Cushing-Gigli saw
  DePuy femoral acetabular overlay
  drill

guide *(cont.)*
  Duopress
  eccentric drill
  FIN pin
  Fisher
  Gigli saw
  Hewson cruciate
  Hewson drill
  Hoffman pin
  intercondylar drill
  long axial alignment
  nail rotational
  neutral drill
  PCA cutting
  PCA medullary
  Synthes wire
  T-bar
  tibial cutting
  tube
guide bushing
guide pin
  ball-point
  ball-tip
  calibrated
guide wire (see *wire)*
Guilford cervical brace
Guillain-Barré syndrome
Guilland sign
Guleke-Stookey approach
Guller resection
gun
  cement
  Harris cement
  staple
Gunning splint
gurney
Gustilio classification of puncture
  wounds
gutter
Guttmann arthrodesis
guy suture
Guyon tunnel release; canal
Gypsona cast material

# H, h

HA 65101 implant metal
Haacker sling
Haas paralysis
hacksaw
Haddad-Riordan arthrodesis
Hagie sliding nail plate
Haglund deformity
Haines-McDougall medial sesamoid ligament
Haldeman bone graft
Hall air-driven oscillating saw
Hallister heel cup
hallux abductovalgus (abductus valgus)
hallux extensus
hallux malleus
hallux nail
hallux rigidus
hallux valgus interphalangeus angle
hallux valgus-metatarsus primus varus complex
hallux varus correction, Johnson-Spiegl
halo, Twin Cities Lo-Profile
halter
   Cerva Crane
   DePuy
   Diskard head
   Forrester-Brown head
   head
   Redi head
   Repro head
   Upper 7 head
   Zimfoam head
   Zimmer head
hamartoma, cartilaginous
Hamas prosthesis
hamate bone, hook of
Hamilton bandage; screw; traction
hammer, Cloward
hammertoe (hammer toe)
Hammond splint
hamstring muscle
hand
   clawhand

hand *(cont.)*
   cleft
   lobster-claw
   mirror
   Myobock
   opera-glass
   psychoextended
   psychoflexed
hand prosthesis (see *prosthesis*)
Hand-Schüller-Christian disease
handbreadth(s)
handle
   Bard-Parker
   Beaver blade
   cup holder
   multisided blade
   surgical knife
Handy-Buck traction
hangup
Hanna night splint
Hansen classification of fractures
Hansen-Street driver-extractor
Hapad medial arch pad
hardware, orthopedic
Hardy-Joyce triangle
Hare device; pin; traction
Harlow plate
Harmon procedure; technique
harness
   figure 8
   Pavlik
   weight-relieving Forte
Harrington rod to correct scoliosis
Harris (HD-2) hip prosthesis
Harris hip scale; score
Harris-Beath arthrodesis
Harris-CDH hip prosthesis
Harris-Galante hip prosthesis
Harris-Smith cervical fusion
Hart splint
Hass procedure
Hassmann-Brunn-Neer elbow technique
Hastings frame; prosthesis
Hatcher pin
Hauser patellar tendon procedure
Hausted orthopedic bed

haversian canal; gland
Hawkins line; sign
Hayes retractor
Haygarth node
Haynes-Stellite 21 (HS-21) implant metal
HD II (or HD 2) total hip prosthesis
head
   Series-II humeral
   terminal
head halter (see *halter*)
headrest extension
heat application
heave, parasternal
Heberden node
Hedley-Hungerford hip prosthesis
heel
   anterior
   black-dot
   painful
   prominent
   rubber walking
   SACH orthopedic
   Thomas
   walking
Heelbo decubitus heel/elbow protector
heel cup (see *cup*)
Heffington lumbar seat spinal frame
Heifetz procedure
Helbing sign
Helenca binder; bandage
Heliodorus bandage
heloma durum
heloma molle
hemangioma
hemangioma, cavernous
hemangiomatosis
hemarthrosis
hematogenous osteomyelitis
hematoma, subungual
hemiarthroplasty (see *operation*)
   Bateman
   I-Beam hip
hemichondrodiasthesis
hemiknee, Savastano
hemilaminectomy
hemimelia, paraxial
hemiparetic
hemipelvis
hemiplegia, hemiplegic
hemivertebra
   balanced
   unbalanced
hemogenesis
hemophilia A
hemophilia B
hemophilia, classic
hemophiliac
hemostasis
hemostat, mosquito
Hemovac suction tube; drain
Henderson onlay graft
Hennessy knee brace
Henry acromioclavicular technique
Henry, master knot of
Henry-Geist spinal fusion technique
Henschke-Mauch SNS knee prosthesis
heparinized Ringer's lactate solution
Herbert knee prosthesis; saw
Hercules plaster shears
herniated nucleus pulposus (HNP)
herniation
   central
   intraspongy nuclear disk
herpetic whitlow (aseptic felon)
Herzmark frame
heterogenesis
heterogeneous, heterogenous
heterotopic ossification
Heuter-Volkmann law
Hewson cruciate guide; button
Hexcel total condylar knee system
Hexcelite cast
Hey-Groves ligament reconstruction technique
Hey-Groves-Kirk bone graft
Heyman-Herndon-Strong technique
hiatus, popliteal
Hibbs spinal fusion technique
Hibbs-Jones spinal fusion procedure
Hibiclens scrub; solution
Hicks lugged plate

Hilgenreiner horizontal Y line
Hilgenreiner-Pauwels line
Hilgenreiner-Perkins line
Hill-Nahai-Vasconez-Mathes technique
Hill-Rom orthopedic bed
Hill-Sach shoulder lesion
Hillock arch
hilum, hilar
hinge
    Arizona Health Sciences Center-Volz
    Bahler
    Dee elbow
    flail-elbow
    kinematic rotating
    Kudo
    Lacey
    Noiles
    Quengel
    stabilizing
hip bump
hip orthosis (see *orthosis*)
hip pointer
hip prosthesis (see *prosthesis*)
hip replacement (see *prosthesis*)
hip skid
hip, hanging
Hippocrates manipulation; bandage
Hirschberg sign
Hirschtick splint
His-Haas muscle transfer
histiocytoma
    angiomatoid
    fibrous
    malignant fibrous
histiocytosis X group of diseases
Hitchcock tendon technique
Hittenberger halo extension
HKAFO (hip-knee-ankle-foot orthosis)
HLA-B27
HNP (herniated nucleus pulposus)
Hoaglund bone graft
Hodgen splint
Hodgkin tumor
Hoen clamp; retractor; skull plate
Hoffer-Daimler cast spreader

Hoffman external fixation
Hoffman-Vidal double frame
Hoffmann sign
Hogg chair
Hohl tibia condylar fracture classification
Hohmann retractor
Hoke lumbar brace/corset
Hoke-Martin traction
holder
    acetabular cup
    arm
    Böhler-Steinmann pin
    bone
    cup
    knee
    leg
    microneedle
    needle
    operative leg
    Schmidt rod
    staple
    tibial track
    well leg
    Zollinger leg
Holdsworth classification
hole
    acetabular seating
    anchoring
    bur
    centering
    drill
    guide
    offset drill
hollow mill Asnis cannulated screw
Hollywood bed extension hook set
Holscher root retractor
Holt bolt; nail; plate
Homans sign
homogeneous graft
homologous graft
hood
    dorsal
    extensor
    retinacular

hook
- Acufex nerve
- APRL (Army Prosthetics Research Laboratory) prosthetic
- Barr
- bone
- distraction
- garment
- Graham nerve
- Harrington
- Leatherman
- meniscus
- prosthetic
- skin
- T-handled
- Trautman Locktite prosthetic
- Zuelzer

Hook hemiharness shoulder immobilizer
hook of hamate bone
Hoppenfeld-Deboer technique
horn
- anterior
- central
- posterior

horseshoe appearance
Horsley bone cutter; saw
Horwitz-Adams arthrodesis
hose, TED
Houghton-Akroyd fracture technique
housemaid's knee
Houston halo cervical support
Hovnanian procedure
Howard bone block
Howmedica ICS screw
Howmedica Vitallium staple
Howorth-Keillor
H-P (Hilgenreiner-Perkins) line
HPS II hip prosthesis
HS (Haynes-Stellite) implant metal
HSMN III (hereditary sensory motor neuropathy, type III)
Hubbard physical therapy tank
Hubbard plate
Huber transfer of abductor digiti quinti

Huck towel
Huckstep nail
Hudson chuck adapter; brace
Hueter bandage; line; sign
Hughston external rotation recurvatum test
Hughston-Degenhardt reconstruction technique
Hughston-Hauser procedure
Hughston-Jacobson technique
Hughston-Losee jerk test
humeroradial articulation
humeroulnar articulation
humerus, humeral
hump
- buffalo
- dowager's

humpback
Hungerford-Krackow-Kenna knee arthroplasty
Hunter silastic rod; prosthesis
Hunter syndrome
Huntington bone graft
Huntington chorea; sign
Hurler disease
Hydra-Cadence gait control unit
hydrogen peroxide
hydroxyapatite, calcium
hypalgesia
Hypaque contrast media
hyperalgesia
hypercalcemia
hyperdynamic abductor hallucis
hyperemic
hyperesthesia
hyperextension stress
hyperkeratosis
hyperostosis
- ankylosing spinal
- diffuse idiopathic sclerosis (DISH)
- infantile cortical

hyperparathyroidism, brown tumor of
hyperplasia, epiphyseal
hyperplastic
hypertonia, hypertonicity
hypertrophy, hypertrophic

hypesthesia (hypoesthesia)
hypochondriac region
hypoesthesia
hyponychium
hypoparathyroidism
hypophosphatasia
hypoplasia
    cartilage-hair
    skeletal
hypothenar eminence
hypotonia, congenital

# I, i

I&D (incision and drainage)
iatrogenic dural tear
ice application
ICLH double cup arthroplasty
ICS (intercostal space)
idiopathic scoliosis
IDK (internal derangement of the knee)
Ilfeld-Gustafson splint
iliac wing
iliotibial band augmentation
ilium, ilial
Ilizarov leg-lengthening technique
Ilizarov ring; wire
IM (intramedullary) rod
image control
image intensifier (x-ray)
imbalance, muscle
imbricate, imbrication
imbrication, capsular
immediate postsurgical fitting (IPSF)
immobilization
    cast
    Rowe-Zarin shoulder
    sling
immobilize, immobilization

immobilizer
    Hook hemi-harness shoulder
    OEC knee
    Raymond shoulder
    sateen knee
    Westfield acromioclavicular
impacter, Austin Moore
impacter-extractor, Fox
impingement, lateral
implant (see *prosthesis*)
implant metal (see *prosthesis*)
Implast bone cement
in situ pinning
in toto
incise, incision
incision and drainage (I&D)
incision (see also *approach*)
    battledore (racquet-shaped)
    bikini skin
    Bruser
    capsular
    Charnley
    chevron
    Cincinnati
    Cubbins
    Curtin
    curvilinear
    deltoid-splitting
    dorsal linear
    dorsomedial
    double
    DuVries
    fascial-splitting
    fiber-splitting
    fishmouth
    Gaenslen split heel
    H-shaped capsular
    Henderson skin
    Henry
    hockey stick
    J-shaped skin
    Kocher
    L-curved
    L-shaped
    lateral
    lateral utility

incision *(cont.)*
   lazy-S
   longitudinal
   Ludloff
   Mayfield
   medial
   medial parapatellar
   midaxillary line
   oblique
   Ollier
   paramedial
   parapatellar
   posterior
   racquet-shaped (battledore)
   relaxing
   relieving
   S-flap
   S-shaped
   saber-cut
   serpentine
   split
   stab
   T-shaped
   transverse
   U-shaped
   V-shaped
   volar
   Wagner skin
   Watson-Jones
   Y
   Y-shaped
   Z-plasty
   zigzag finger
incisura
Inclan-Ober procedure
incontinence, urinary
incorporation (new-bone formation)
increment
index, indices
   ankle-arm
   Gardens alignment
   McMurtry kinematic
   Singh osteoporosis
Indiana conservative prosthesis
Indong Oh hip prosthesis
indurate, indurated, induration

infarct, bone
infarction, Freiberg
infection
   felon
   pin tract
   INFH (ischemic necrosis of femoral head)
inflame, inflamed, inflammation
inflate, inflated, inflation
infraisthmal
infragluteal crease
infrapatellar tendinitis
infraspinatus tendon
Inge retractor
Inglis-Cooper technique
Inglis-Pellicci elbow arthroplasty rating system
Inglis-Ranawat-Straub technique
Ingram-Bachynski classification of hip fracture
Ingram-Withers-Speltz motor test
ingrowth, bone
inion bump
injection, Black peroneal tendon sheath
injury
   brachial plexus
   contrecoup
   crush
   degloving
   soft tissue
   softball sliding
Inland Super Multi-Hite orthopedic bed
inner table
innominate bone
Insall ligament reconstruction technique
Insall patella alta method
Insall-Burstein semiconstrained tricompartmental knee prosthesis
Insall-Burstein-Freeman knee arthroplasty
Insall-Hood reconstruction technique
insert
   Alimed

insert *(cont.)*
    cushioned shoe
    NYU (New York University) orthosis
    Poly-Dial
    polypropylene
    silicone gel socket
    sole
    Spanko shoe
inserter
    C-wire
    CDH cup
    cerclage wire
    Kirschner wire
    Massie
    staple
    T-shaped
inserter-extractor, compression
insertion
    anomalous
    Bosworth bone peg
    percutaneous pin
insidious
instability
    anterolateral rotary knee
    dorsal intercalary segment (DISI)
    joint
    rotational
instrument, sponge, and needle
    count(s)
instrumentation
    Dwyer spinal
    Harrington
    hollow mill
    Howmedica knee
    McElroy
    Putti-Platt
    Zielke
insufflate, insufflated
intact
    neurologically
    neurovascularly
intensifier, image (x-ray)
Inter-Royal frame orthopedic bed
intercarpal articulation
intercondylar notch
intercostal space (ICS)

intercostobrachial nerve
interdigital ligament
interface
    acetabular-prosthetic
    bone-cement
    bony
    cement
    implant-cement
intergluteal cleft
interlaminar
intermetacarpal articulation
intermetatarsal angle
intermuscular septum
internal rotation in extension (IRE)
internal rotation in flexion (IRF)
interosseous membrane
interpediculate
interphalangeal articulation
interposition, interpositioned
interposition, soft tissue
intertrigo
interspace
interspinous pseudarthrosis
interstices, bone
interstitial meniscal tear
intertrochanteric plate
intervention, nonsurgical
intervertebral disk narrowing
intoeing
intra-acetabular
intra-articular loose body
intracapsular osteotomy
Intracath needle
intracompartmental ischemia and
    edema
intracortical osteogenic sarcoma
intracuticular stitch
intradermal suture
intramedullary rod
intramuscular injection
intraoperative complications
intraosseous venography
intraprosthetic
intratendinous
intrinsic minus deformity (clawhand)
intrinsic minus hallux

intrinsic plus deformity
intrinsics, finger
invagination
invert, inversion
invertors
involucrum
iodoform gauze
iodophor solution
Iohexol contrast media
Iowa internal prosthesis
IPSF (immediate postsurgical fitting)
ipsilateral
IRE (internal rotation in extension)
IRF (internal rotation in flexion)
iridocyclitis
iron, Jewett bending
irreducible fracture
irrigating (irrigation) solution
irrigation of wound
irrigator
   jet
   ophthalmic
   pulse
irritability, nerve root
ischemia
   intracompartmental
   muscle
   Volkmann
ischial tuberosity
ischiogluteal bursa
ischium, ischial
Ishizuki unconstrained elbow
   prosthesis
island, bone (bony)
Israel retractor
isthmus
IT (iliotibial) band
ITT (internal tibial torsion)

*Iron knee brace*

# J, j

J sign
J-shaped skin incision
Jaboulay amputation
jacket
   flexion body
   Frejka
   halo body
   Kydex body
   Minerva cervical
   orthoplast
   Royalite body
   von Lackum transection shift
   Wilmington
Jackson-Pratt drain
Jacobs chuck adapter
Jaffe disease; procedure
Jaffe-Capello-Averill hip prosthesis
Jamar dynamometer; grip tester
Janes frame
Jansen test
Jansey technique
Japas V-osteotomy
Jarcho-Levin syndrome
Jefferson fracture
Jeffery classification of radial fracture
Jelanko splint
Jendrassik maneuver
Jenet sign
Jergesen I-beam; plate
jerk
   ankle
   knee
   patellar
jet, Ortholav
Jewett bending iron; brace; plate
jig
   chamfer cut
   drilling
   femoral alignment
   Miller-Galante
   spacer-tensor
   tibial
Jobst stocking; brassiere

Joerns orthopedic bed
Johannesberg staple
Johannson lag screw
John C. Wilson arthrodesis
Johnson-Spiegl hallux varus correction
Johnson-Zuck-Wingate motor test
joint
   AC (acromioclavicular)
   atlantoaxial
   bail-lock knee
   ball-and-socket
   calcaneocuboid
   carpometacarpal
   Charcot
   Chopart
   costovertebral
   cuneiform
   DIP (distal interphalangeal)
   ellipsoid
   facet
   flail
   free knee
   glenohumeral
   gliding
   hinge
   hip capsule
   immovable
   Lisfranc
   Luschka
   MCP, MP (metacarpophalangeal)
   metatarsocuneiform
   MTP (metatarsophalangeal)
   PIP (proximal interphalangeal)
   pivot
   sacroiliac (SI)
   saddle
   SI (sacroiliac)
   sternoclavicular
   subtalar
   synovial
   talonavicular
   tarsometatarsal
   tibiofibular
   tibiotalar
   uncovertebral
   weightbearing

Joint Jack finger splint
joint line tenderness
joint position sense (JPS)
joint stiffness
joint swelling
joint warmth
Jonell splint
Jones compression plate
Jones, Carl P., traction splint
Jones-Brackett technique
Joplin toe prosthesis
Joseph splint
JPS (joint position sense)
JRA (juvenile rheumatoid arthritis)
J.R. Moore procedure
Jude pelvic x-ray
Judet graft
Judet hip prosthesis
Judet hip status system
jumper's knee position
junction, meniscosynovial
junctura
jury-rig
juxta-articulation
juxtacortical chondroma

juddering

# K, k

K pack
K pad
K wire (Kirschner wire)
K-wire skeletal traction
K-F (Kayser-Fleischer) ring)
Kaessmann nail; screw
KAFO (knee-ankle-foot orthosis)
Kager triangle
Kampe corset
Kanavel cock-up splint
Kapel elbow dislocation technique
Kaplan technique
Karakousis-Vezeridis resection

*Kegel exercises*

Karfoil splint
Kashiwagi technique
Kate procedure
Kates-Kessel-Kay technique
Kaufer tendon technique
Kayser-Fleischer (K-F) ring
Kazanjian splint
keel of glenoid component
Keen sign
Keith needle
Kelikian-Clayton-Loseff technique
Kelikian-McFarland procedure
Kelikian-Riashi-Gleason technique
Keller-Blake half-ring splint
Kellgren sign
Kellogg-Speed lumbar spinal fusion
Kelly clamp; forceps
keloid
Ken driver-extractor; nail
Kendrick-Sharma-Hassler-Herndon technique
Kennedy ligament technique
Kenny Howard shoulder sling
keratosis, plantar
Kerlix dressing; wrap
Kern bone-holding forceps
Kernig sign
Kerr sign; splint
Kerr-Lagen abdominal support
Kerrison curet; punch; rongeur
Kessel-Bonney extension osteotomy
Kessler prosthesis; suture; traction
Ketac cement
Key intra-articular knee arthrodesis
key the cement
Key-Conwell classification of pelvic fracture
keyhole tenodesis technique
Keys-Kirschner traction
keystone of the calcar arch
keyway
Kickaldy-Willis arthrodesis
Kidner procedure for accessory navicular
kidney rest
Kienböck disease (lunatomalacia)

Kilfoyle classification of condylar fracture
Kimura disease
Kinematic Howmedica
kinematic indices of McMurtry
King intra-articular hip fusion
King traction; brace
King-Richards dislocation technique
King-Steelquist technique
Kirner deformity
Kirschner Medical Dimension hip replacement
Kirschner wire (K wire)
Kite clubfoot casting
Kjolbe technique
Klein approach; technique
Kleinert repair
Klengall brace
Klenzak spring brace
Klinefelter syndrome
Kling elastic bandage
Klippel-Feil syndrome
Klippel-Trenaunay syndrome
Klisic-Jankovic technique
Klumpke palsy
knee
  anterior cruciate deficit
  breaststroker's
  dislocated
  hamstrung
  housemaid's
  jumper's
  locked
  runner's
knee brace (see *brace*)
knee immobilizer (see *immobilizer*)
knee orthosis (see *orthosis*)
knee prosthesis (see *prosthesis*)
kneecap
knife (blade)
  acetabular
  amputation
  arthroscopic
  banana
  Bard-Parker
  Beaver-DeBakey
  Cotrel-Dubousset

knife *(cont.)*
  Blount
  Bovie
  cartilage
  chondroplasty
  Downing cartilage
  Freiberg meniscectomy
  full-radius resector
  hemilaminectomy
  hot
  Krull acetabular
  Lowe-Breck meniscectomy
  Oretorp arthroscopy
  Ridlon plaster
  Smillie meniscus
  Smillie-Beaver
  tenotomy
  Weck
Knight back brace
Knight-Taylor thoracic brace
Knobby-Clark procedure
knock-knee (genu valgum) deformity
Knodt rod
knot, Henry
Knowles nail; pin
knuckle-shaped
Koch-Mason dressing
Kocher lateral J approach
Kocher-McFarland hip arthroplasty
Kodel knee sling
Koenig-Schaefer approach
Köhler disease
Koutsogiannis-Fowler-Anderson osteotomy
Krackow point
Kramer-Craig-Noel osteotomy technique
Krempen-Craig-Sotelo tibia nonunion technique
Kreuscher bunionectomy
Kristiansen eyelet lag screw
Kronner external fixation
Krukenberg operation
Krull acetabular knife
Kudo unconstrained elbow prosthesis
Kugelberg-Welander disease

Kuhlmann traction
Kumar spica cast technique
Kumar-Cowell-Ramsey technique
Kümmell disease
Küntscher nail; pin
Kurtzke score (multiple sclerosis)
Kutler V-Y flap graft
Kydex body jacket
kyphectomy, Sharrard-type
kyphoscoliosis
kyphosis
  lumbar
  lumbosacral
  Scheuermann juvenile
kyphotic

# L, l

L plate
L-shaped incision
L-spine (lumbar spine)
L1 to L6 intervertebral disks
labium
labrum
  acetabular
  articular
  glenoid
LAC (long arm cast)
laceration
  bursting-type
  chevron
  stellate
Lacey knee prosthesis
Lachman maneuver; test
lacunae
Lahey clamp
Laing concentric hip cup
Lamb muscle transfer
lamb's wool pad
Lambert-Lowman bone clamp
Lambrinudi operation; splint

lamella | 69 | Leri

lamella, lamellae, lamellar
lamellae, concentric
laminaplasty, Tsuji
laminectomy, decompression
laminectomy frame
laminotomy
lamp, Wood
landmark, bony
Landouzy-Dejerine disease
Landsmeer ligament
Lane bone-holding forceps
Lanex screen
Lange tendon lengthening and repair
Langenbeck periosteal elevator
Langenskiöld bony bridge resection
Langer line
Langoria sign
lap (laparotomy) sponge
laparotomy sheet
Lapidus bunionectomy
Larmon forefoot procedure
Larson ligament reconstruction
Lasègue sign; test
lateral head of gastrocnemius
lateralization
latissimus dorsi
latticework
Lauge-Hansen classification of ankle fracture
Laugier sign
lavage
    Exeter bone
    jet
    joint
    pulsatile pressure
law
    Heuter-Volkmann
    von Schwann
    Wolff
Lawson-Thornton plate
laxity, ligamentous
laxity of ligament
laxity to varus stress
layer, periosteal cambium
LCL (lateral collateral ligament)
LCP (Legg-Calve-Perthes disease)

LCS New Jersey knee prosthesis
Le Fort fibular fracture
Le Fort mandible fracture
LE prep (lupus erythematosus preparation)
Leach-Igou step-cut medial osteotomy
Leadbetter maneuver
leaf
    inferior
    superior
Leatherman hook
Lee bone graft
left-hand dominant
leg holder (see *holder*)
leg
    badger
    baker
    bandy
    bayonet
    bow
    game
    rider's
    scissor
    tennis
Legg-Calve-Perthes disease (LCP)
Legg-Perthes sling; shoe extension
Lehman technique
Leichtenstern sign
Leinbach femoral prosthesis
leiomyosarcoma
Leksell rongeur
Lenart-Kullman technique
lengthening
    Achilles tendon
    Armistead ulnar
    gastrocnemius
    Ilizarov leg
    Tachdjian hamstring
    tendon
    Vulpius
    Vulpius-Compere Z
Lenox Hill derotational knee brace
L'Episcopo-Zachary procedure
leptomeninges
Leri sign

Lerman multiligamentous knee control
    orthosis
lesion
    Bankart shoulder
    cleavage
    desmoid
    Hill-Sach shoulder
    Kidner
    lytic bone
Letournel plate
Letterer-Siwe disease
Leung thumb loss classification
level of activity
levering
Levis splint
levoscoliosis
Lewin baseball-finger splint
Lewin-Stern splint
Lewis-Chekofsky resection
Lhermitte sign
Lichtman technique
Liebolt radioulnar technique
lifestyle, sedentary
lift, DiPalma shoe
ligament
    accessory collateral
    acromioclavicular
    acromiocoracoid
    annular
    anterior collateral (ACL)
    anterior cruciate
    atlantal
    calcaneonavicular
    capsular
    check
    Cleland
    collateral
    congenital laxity of
    coracoacromial
    coracoclavicular
    coracohumeral
    cruciate
    deep collateral
    Gerdy
    Grayson
    Haines-McDougall medial
ligament *(cont.)*
    inferior ilioischial
    intercarpal
    interdigital
    interspinous
    Landsmeer
    lateral collateral (LCL)
    medial collateral (MCL)
    meniscotibial
    natatory
    nuchal
    posterior cruciate
    posterior longitudinal
    posterior oblique (POL)
    Poupart inguinal
    radioscaphoid
    sacrotuberous
    Struthers
    tibiofibular
    torn meniscotibial
    triangular
    vaginal hand
    Wrisberg
ligamentoplasty
ligamentous bouncing
ligamentum flavum
ligamentum teres
light conductor, Bozzini
light source, fiberoptic
limb absence
    congenital intercalary
    congenital terminal
limbus annularis
limitation of joint motion
limp
Lindeman procedure
Linder sign
Lindholm technique
line
    bisector
    Blumensaat
    Chamberlain
    epiphyseal
    fracture
    Fränkle white
    growth arrest

line *(cont.)*
  H-P (Hilgenreiner-Perkins)
  Harris
  Hawkins
  Hilgenreiner horizontal Y
  Hilgenreiner-Pauwels
  Hilgenreiner-Perkins (H-P)
  Hueter
  joint
  Langer
  lateral joint
  lead
  McGregor
  medial joint
  Nélaton
  nipple
  Perkins
  Shenton
  Wineberger
  Zahn
linea aspera
Ling hip prosthesis
lip of acetabulum
lip of glenoid
lipoblastomatosis
lipochondrodystrophy
lipofibroma
lipoma
liposarcoma
  myxoid-type
  pleomorphic
  round cell type
lipping
Lippman hip prosthesis
Lipscomb modified McKeever arthrodesis
Lisfranc below-knee prosthesis
Lister tubercle
Liston splint
lists to the right (or left)
litter, Neal-Robertson
Little Leaguer's elbow; shoulder
Littler-Cooley transfer of abductor digiti quinti
Liverpool elbow prosthesis

living
  activities of daily (ADLs)
  normal activities of daily
Livingston intramedullary bar
LLC (long leg cast)
LLD (leg length discrepancy)
LLE (left lower extremity)
Lloyd adapter for Smith-Petersen nail
Lloyd-Roberts fracture technique
LLWC (long leg walking cast)
load, torque
loading, axial
Loban adhesive drape
local standby (anesthesia) technique
Localio procedure
Locke elevator
locking of joint
locomotor ataxia
Lofstrand crutch
Logan traction
London unconstrained elbow prosthesis
longstanding
longitudinal blood supply to ulnar nerve
loop, figure-of-8 wire
loop-lock cock-up splint
Loose procedure
Lord hip prosthesis
lordosis
  cervical
  lumbar
  reversal of
  thoracic
Lorenz cast; procedure; sign
Lorenzo screw
Losee modification of MacIntosh technique
loss of motion
loss, sensory
Lottes triflanged medullary nail
Lou Gehrig disease
loupe
  binocular
  magnification
  magnifying
Love root retractor

Lovell     72     *Mal perforans (doofulce)* maneuver

Lovell clubfoot cast
LowDye taping technique
Lowe-Breck meniscectomy knife
Lowe-Miller unconstrained elbow prosthesis
Lowman bone clamp
LS (lumbosacral) spine
LSU (Louisiana State University) reciprocation-gait orthosis
Lucas-Murray knee arthrodesis
lucency, lucent
Luck-Bishop bone saw
Ludloff incision; sign; technique
LUE (left upper extremity)
lumbago
lumbar spine (L1 to L5 or L6)
lumbarization
lumbosacral kyphosis
lumbosacral series (x-rays)
lumbrical bar
lunate dislocation
lunatomalacia (Kienböck disease)
Lunceford-Pilliar-Engh hip prosthesis
Lundholm plate; screw
lupus erythematosus preparation (LE prep)
Luque rod fixation for kyphosis
Luschka bursa
Luschka, joint of
luxated bone
luxatio coxae congenita
luxatio erecta shoulder dislocation
luxatio perinealis
luxation
Lyden-Lehman technique
Lyman-Smith brace; traction
Lyme disease
lymphadenopathy
lymphangiography
lymphedema, familial
lymphoma
Lynn technique
Lyofoam wound dressing
lyophilization (freeze-drying)
lytic bone lesions
Lytle splint

# M, m

MacAusland lumbar brace; procedure
MacCarthy procedure
maceration
MacEwen-Shands osteotomy
machine
   CPM (continuous passive motion)
   Cybex
MacIntosh extra-articular tenodesis
MacIntosh over-the-top ACL reconstruction
MacNab-English shoulder prosthesis
MacNichol-Voutsinas classification
macrodactyly
Madelung deformity
madreporic hip prosthesis
Maffucci syndrome
Magilligan technique for measuring anteversion
magnet, Dyonics Golden Retriever
magnification, loupe
Magnuson-Stack shoulder arthrotomy
Ma-Griffith technique
Maisonneuve fibular fracture
Majestro-Ruda-Frost tendon technique
malalignment
malangulation
Malawer excision technique
Malgaigne pelvic fracture
malleable template
malleolus, malleoli
   lateral
   medial
mallet, bone
malrotation
malum coxae senilis
malunion, malunited
maneuver (see also *reflex; sign; test*)
   Adson
   Allen
   Barlow
   circumduction
   closed manipulative
   flexion-extension

maneuver *(cont.)*
   flexion-rotation-compression
   Fowler
   Hippocratic
   Jendrassik
   Kocher
   Lachman
   Leadbetter
   McMurray circumduction
   Ortolani
   osteoclasis
   Phalen
   postural fixation back
   rotation-compression
   Schreiber
   Slocum
   Valsalva
manipulate
manipulation
   fine
   gross
   Hippocrates
   opening wedge
Mankin technique
Manktelow transfer procedure
Mann modified McKeever arthrodesis
Mann-Coughlin-DuVries cheilectomy
Mann-DuVries arthroplasty
Manske technique
mapping the defect
Maquet procedure; technique
march foot
Marcus-Balourdas-Heiple ankle fusion technique
Marfan syndrome
margo
Marie-Bamberger disease
Marie-Charcot-Tooth disease
Marie-Foix sign
Marie-Strümpell disease
Marion screw
marker, skin
Markham-Meyerding retractor
Marks-Bayne technique for thumb duplication
Marmor modular knee prosthesis

Maroteaux-Lamy syndrome
marrow
   red
   yellow
Marshall ligament repair technique
marshmallows
Martin patellar wiring technique
Mason-Allen universal splint
Massie sliding nail *(not* massive)
MAST (medical antishock trousers)
master knot of Henry
Matchett-Brown internal prosthesis
matchsticked
material
   Plasti-Pore prosthetic
   Porocoat prosthetic
   porous prosthetic material
   Proplast prosthetic
matricectomy, phenol
matrix
   germinal
   nail
Matti-Russe technique
mattress, eggcrate
maturity, skeletal
Mauck procedure
MaxCast casting tape
Maxon suture
Mayer splint
Mayfield incision
Mayo semiconstrained elbow prosthesis
Mayo-Collins retractor
Mazas totally constrained elbow prosthesis
Mazet technique
Mazur ankle rating system
McKee-Farrar total hip prosthesis
McLaughlin plate
McReynolds driver-extractor
McBride bunionectomy
McBride femoral prosthesis
McCarroll-Baker procedure
McConnell technique
McElfresh-Dobyns-O'Brien technique
McElroy instrumentation
McFarland-Osborne technique

McGee splint
McGregor line
McIntire splint
McKee totally constrained elbow prosthesis
McKee-Farrar acetabular cup
McKeever-Buck elbow technique
McKeever Vitallium knee prosthesis
MCL (medial collateral ligament)
McLaughlin modification of Bunnell pull-out suture
McLaughlin nail; plate; screw
McLaughlin-Hay technique
McLeod splint
McMaster bone graft
McMurray maneuver for torn knee cartilage
McMurtry, kinematic indices of
MCP (metacarpophalangeal) joint
McReynolds open reduction technique
McWhorter shoulder approach
MD (muscular dystrophy)
Mears sacroiliac plate
measurement
  Schober
  skin fluorescence
  tissue pressure
mechanics, body
mechanism
  extensor
  extensor hood
  flexor
  quadriceps
  tendo Achillis
  Windlass
medialization
medications
  A-hydroCort (hydrocortisone)
  A-methaPred (methylprednisolone)
  acetaminophen
  acetylsalicylic acid (ASA, aspirin)
  allopurinol
  Alpha Chymar (alpha-chymotrypsin)
  alpha-chymotrypsin
  alprazolam
  ampicillin

medications *(cont.)*
  Ancef (cefazolin)
  anti-inflammatory
  Anturane (sulfinpyrazone)
  ASA (acetylsalicylic acid, aspirin)
  Ascriptin (aspirin)
  aspirin
  atracurium besylate
  auranofin
  aurothioglucose
  baclofen
  Benemid (probenecid)
  bupivacaine
  Cama (aspirin)
  carisoprodol
  carprofen
  cefazolin
  chlorzoxazone
  choline magnesium trisalicylate
  chymopapain
  Clinoril (sulindac)
  ColBenemid (probenecid)
  corticosteroid
  cortisone
  Cortone (cortisone)
  Cuprimine (penicillamine)
  cyclobenzaprine
  Dantrium (dantrolene)
  dantrolene
  Deltasone (prednisone)
  Depo-Medrol (methylprednisolone)
  dexamethasone
  diazepam
  Didronel (etidronate)
  dihydrocodeine
  Elase
  Elase-Chloromycetin ointment
  Empirin with codeine
  Equagesic (meprobamate)
  etidronate
  Excedrin
  Feldene (piroxicam)
  fenoprofen
  ferrous sulfate (FeSO$_4$, iron)
  Flexeril (cyclobenzaprine)
  Furacin (nitrofurazone)

medications *(cont.)*
  gold salts
  gold sodium thiomalate
  Hexadrol (dexamethasone)
  hydrocodone
  hydrocortisone
  Hydrocortone (hydrocortisone)
  ibuprofen
  Kantrex (kanamycin)
  Kefzol (cefazolin)
  Lioresal (baclofen)
  Lopurin (allopurinol)
  Marcaine (bupivacaine)
  meclofenamate
  Meclomen (meclofenamate)
  Medipren (ibuprofen)
  Medrol Dosepak
  metaxalone
  methocarbamol
  methylprednisolone
  Monocid (cefonicid)
  Motrin (ibuprofen)
  muscle relaxant
  Myochrysine (gold sodium thiomalate)
  Nalfon (fenoprofen)
  Naprosyn (naproxen)
  Neosporin ointment
  nitrofurazone
  nonsteroidal anti-inflammatory
  Norflex (orphenadrine)
  Norgesic (orphenadrine)
  NSAID (nonsteroidal anti-inflammatory drug)
  orphenadrine
  oxycodone
  oxyphenbutazone
  Panadol (acetaminophen)
  Paraflex (chlorzoxazone)
  Parafon Forte (chlorzoxazone)
  Percocet (oxycodone)
  Percodan (oxycodone)
  Percogesic (acetaminophen)
  piroxicam
  Predate S
  Prednicen-M (prednisone)

medications *(cont.)*
  prednisolone
  prednisone
  probenecid
  Ridaura (auranofin)
  Rimadyl (carprofen)
  Robaxin (methocarbamol)
  Robaxisal (methocarbamol)
  Skelaxin (metaxalone)
  Solganal (aurothioglucose)
  Solu-Cortef (hydrocortisone)
  Solu-Medrol (methylprednisolone)
  Soma (carisoprodol)
  sulfinpyrazone
  sulindac
  suprofen
  Suprol (suprofen)
  Synalgos-DC (dihydrocodeine)
  Tandearil (oxyphenbutazone)
  Tolectin DS (tolmetin)
  tolmetin
  Tracium (atracurium besylate)
  Trilisate (choline magnesium trisalicylate)
  Tylenol (acetaminophen)
  Tylox (oxycodone)
  Valium (diazepam)
  Valrelease (diazepam)
  Vicodin (hydrocodone)
  Xanax (alprazolam)
  Xylocaine (lidocaine)
  Zyloprim (allopurinol)
medicine, sports
Mediloy implant metal
mediolateral stress
Medipedic Multicentric knee brace
medulla, medullary
Meek clavicle strap
meglumine diatrizoate contrast media
melorheostosis
membrane
  basement
  interosseous
  synovial
  thickened synovial
Mendel-Bekhterev reflex; sign

meningioma
meningism
meningismus
meningitis
meningocele
meningoencephalomyelitis
meningomyelitis
meningomyelocele
meniscal tear (see *tear*)
meniscectomy
   arthroscopic
   partial
   Patel medial
   subtotal lateral
   total
meniscitis
meniscosynovial junction
meniscotibial ligament
meniscotome, Bowen-Grover
meniscal
meniscus, menisci
   discoid
   lateral
   medial
   torn
Mennell sign
Mensor-Scheck technique
meralgia paresthetica
Merchant angle
Mersilene suture; tape
mesenchymal chondrosarcoma
mesenchymoma, pluripotential
mesh, metal
mesotenon
metacarpophalangeal (MCP or MP)
   dislocation; joint
metacarpus, metacarpal
metal locator, Berman-Moorhead
metal (see *implant metal*)
metaphyseal-epiphyseal angle
metaphysis, distal
metaplasia
   cartilaginous
   osteocartilaginous
metatarsal neck osteotomy
metatarsalgia

metatarsocuneiform joint
metatarsophalangeal (MTP) joint
metatarsus abductus (MTA)
metatarsus primus varus (MPV)
metatarsus varus (MTV)
meter, pinch
method
   Abbott
   Bleck
   Borggreve
   Budin-Chandler
   Cobb
   Ferguson scoliosis measuring
   hydrogen washout
   Insall patella alta
methylene blue
methyl methacrylate cement
methyl methacrylate, centrifuged
metrizamide contrast media
Metzenbaum scissors
Meurig Williams plate
Meyerding chisel; osteotome; gouge
Meyerding-Van Demark technique
Meyers-McKeever classification of
   tibial fracture
Meynet node
mice, joint
Michael Reese articulated prosthesis
Michel clip
Micro-Aire debridement of bone
   surfaces
micro-pin, Pischel
microcirculation
microcurrent therapy
Microfoam dressing
microscissors
microscope, double binocular operating
Midas Rex pneumatic instruments
midaxillary line incision
midcalf
Middeldorpf splint; triangle
midfemur
midfoot
midpatellar tendon
midshaft fracture
midthigh

migration of acetabular cup
Mik pad
Mikhail bone block
Mikulicz angle; pad; sponge
Milch cuff resection of ulna technique
milking of vessel
Milkman syndrome
Millender-Nalebuff wrist arthrodesis
Miller-Galante knee arthroplasty
Millesi modified technique
millimeters of mercury (mmHg)
milling-cutter
Mills test
Milroy disease
Milwaukee cervicothoracolumbosacral orthosis
mimocausalgia
mineralization
Minerva cast; jacket
Minneapolis prosthesis
Minor sign
Mira reamer
misshapen
Mital elbow release technique
Mitchell osteotomy
Mittlemeier noncemented femoral prosthesis; broach
MixEvac bone-cement mixer
Mizuno technique
mmHg (millimeters of mercury)
Moberg-Gedda open reduction, fracture
mobile, mobility
mobility, joint
modification (see *operation*)
Modny pin
modulus of elasticity
Moe modified Cotrel cast; plate
Mohr splint
mold, Aufranc concentric hip
Molesworth-Campbell elbow approach
monarticular
Mönckeberg sclerosis
monitoring, fluorescein perfusion
Monk hip prosthesis
monoclonal gammopathy

Monteggia fracture-dislocation of ulna
Montercaux fracture
Monticelli-Spinelli distraction technique
Montreal hip positioner
Moon Boot brace; shoe
Mooney brace; cast
Moore osteotomy-osteoclasis
Moore stem
mooring
morcellation, Robinnson-Chung-Farahvar clavicular
Moreira bolt; plate
Morel syndrome
Morgan-Casscells meniscus suturing technique
Morquio sign; syndrome
Morrey-Bryan total elbow arthroplasty
Morris biphase screw
Morrison technique
Morse tapered prosthetic post
mortise, ankle
mortise, mortised
Morton foot; neuroma; sign; test
Morton-Horwitz nerve cross-over sign
Moseley straight line graph
motion
  arc of
  limitation of
  scapulothoracic
motor activity
Mouradian rod; screw
mouse, joint
MP (or MCP) joint (metacarpophalangeal)
MP35N implant metal prosthesis
MPV (metatarsus primus varus)
MS (multiple sclerosis)
MST-6A1-4V implant metal prosthesis
MT or MTP (metatarsophalangeal) joint
MTA (metatarsus adductus)
MTV (metatarsus varus)
Mubarak-Hargens decompression technique
mucopolysaccharides

mucopolysaccharidosis
Mueli wrist prosthesis
Müller dual-lock hip prosthesis
Müller plate; wrench
multangular
   greater
   lesser
multiple sclerosis (MS)
Mumford-Gurd arthroplasty
Murphy-Lane bone skid
Murray-Jones splint
Murray-Thomas splint
muscle, musculi
muscle belly
muscle-plasty, Speed V-Y
muscle relaxant
muscle-setting exercises
muscular atrophy
muscular dystrophy (MD)
   Becker
   Duchenne
musculoskeletal trauma
musculotendinous junction
MWD (microwave diathermy)
myalgia
myasthenia gravis
myatrophy
mycopolysaccharidosis
myectomy
myelalgia
myelanalosis
myelasthenia
myelatelia
myelatrophy
myelauxe
myeleterosis
myeloblastoma
myelocele
myelocystocele
myelocystomeningocele
myelodiastasis
myelodysplasia
myelofibrosis
myelogram
myelolipoma
myeloma, multiple

myeloma, plasma cell
myelomalacia
myelomeningocele
myeloneuritis
myeloparalysis
myelopathy, cervical
myelophthisis
myeloplegia
myeloradiculitis
myeloradiculopathy
myelorrhaphy, commissural
myelotomy
Myers knee retractor
myoasthenia
myoblast
myoblastoma, granular cell
Myobock artificial hand
myobradia
myocele
myocelialgia
myocelitis
myocerosis
myocervical collar
myoclasis
myoclonia
myoclonus
myocoele
myocytoma
myodegeneration
myodemia
myodesis
myodiastasis
myodynia
myodystonia
myoedema
myofasciitis
myofibril
myofibroma
myofibrosis
myofibrositis
myogelosis
myohypertrophia
myoischemia
myokerosis
myolipoma
myolysis

myoma
myomalacia
myomatosis
myomectomy (myomatectomy)
myomelanosis
myoneuralgia
myoneurasthenia
myoneurectomy
myoneuroma
myoneurosis
myopachynsis
myopalmus
myoparalysis
myoparesis
myopathy, steroid
myophagism
myoplasty
myopsychopathy
myorrhaphy
myorrhexis
myosalgia
myosarcoma
myosclerosis
myoseism
myositis
  ischemic
  ossificans
  proliferative
myositis fibrosa
myositis ossificans progressiva
myospamia
myospasia
myospasm
myosteoma
myosynizesis
myotenontoplasty
myotenotomy
myotomy
myotonia intermittens
myotonia, congenital
mytenositis
myxofibroma
myxoma, soft tissue
myxosarcoma

# N, n

Naffziger sign; syndrome
nail (see also *nailing)*
  adjustable
  AO slotted medullary
  AP
  Augustine boat
  Bailey-Dubow
  Barr
  boat
  Brooker femoral
  Brooker-Willis
  cannulated
  Chick
  Christensen interlocking
  cloverleaf Küntscher
  Curry hip
  diamond-shaped medullary
  Dooley
  dynamic locking
  Enders flexible medullary
  Engel-May
  four-flanged
  Grosse-Kempf interlocking
    medullary
  hallux
  Hansen-Street
  Harris medullary
  Holt
  hooked intramedullary
  Huckstep
  ingrown (onychocryptosis)
  interlocking
  intramedullary
  Jewett
  Kaessmann
  Ken
  Ken sliding
  Knowles
  Küntscher
  left-sided
  Lottes triflanged medullary
  Massie II *(not* massive)
  Massie sliding *(not* massive)

nail *(cont.)*
  McKee tri-fin
  McLaughlin
  medullary
  Moore
  nested
  Neufeld
  noncannulated
  Nylok self-locking
  PGP
  Pitcock
  prebent
  Pugh sliding
  right-sided
  Rush flexible medullary
  Russell-Taylor interlocking
    medullary
  Sage triangular
  Sampson medullary
  Sarmiento
  Schneider medullary
  self-broaching
  self-locking
  Slocum
  Smillie
  Smith-Petersen transarticular
  static locking
  Street
  telescoping
  Temple University
  Thatcher
  Thornton
  Tiemann
  triangular medullary
  triflange
  triflanged Lottes
  V-medullary
  Venable-Stuck
  Vesely-Street split
  Vitallium Küntscher
  Watson-Jones
  Webb
  Z fixation
  Zickel subtrochanteric
  Zickel supracondylar medullary
nail assembly, Massie
nail bed
nailing (see also *nail)*
  blind medullary
  closed
  closed Küntscher
  condylocephalic
  crutch and belt femoral closed
  Ender
  Grosse-Kempf interlocking
    medullary
  Harris condylocephalic
  Küntscher medullary
  open
nail starter, Ritchie
Nalebuff-Millender technique
natatory ligament
Naughton-Dunn triple arthrodesis
Nauth traction apparatus
navicular cookie in shoe
navicular, accessory
naviculocapitate fracture syndrome
NCV (nerve conduction velocity)
Neal-Robertson litter
NEB (New England Baptist)
NEB hip prosthesis
neck
  basal
  supple
  surgical
necrosis
  aseptic
  avascular
  epiphyseal ischemic
  gangrenous
  ischemic n. of femoral head (INFH)
  septic
  skin
necrotizing fasciitis
needle
  Beath
  bone biopsy
  bore
  Bouge
  Bunnell
  Gallie
  hubbed

needle *(cont.)*
   Intracath
   Keith
   spinal
   tendon
   Verbrugge
needle holder
   Wangensteen
   Webster
Neer acromioplasty for rotator cuff tear
Neer shoulder prosthesis
Neer-Horowitz classification
Neer-Vitallium humeral prosthesis
Nélaton dislocation of ankle
Nélaton line; drain
Nelson finger exerciser
neoplastic disorder
   benign
   malignant
neoprene patellar brace
nerve conduction velocity (NCV)
nerve root compression
nerve separator, Sach
Neubeiser splint
Neufeld cast; nail; screw; traction
Neurairtome
neural arch resection technique
neuralgia
neurapraxia
neurasthenia
neurectomy
neurilemmoma
neuritis
neurofibroma, nonplexiform cutaneous
neurofibromatosis
neurologically intact
neurolysis
neuroma
   amputation
   interdigital
   Morton
neuropathy
   compressive
   hereditary sensory motor (HSMN)
   peripheral

neuroplasty
neurorrhaphy
   epineurial
   perineurial
neurotmesis
neurotomy
neurotripsy
neurovascular impairment
neurovascular status
Neviaser acromioclavicular technique
Neviaser-Wilson-Gardner transfer
New England Baptist (NEB) acetabular cup
New Jersey LCS knee prosthesis
new bone formation (incorporation)
Newington brace; orthosis
Newman classification of radial fracture
Newton ankle prosthesis
newtons of force (SI units)
Nicholas five-in-one reconstruction technique
Nicholas ligament technique
Nicoll cancellous bone graft
Niebauer metacarpophalangeal joint Silastic prosthesis
Niebauer-King technique
Niemann-Pick disease
Ninhydrin print test
Nirschl technique
nitrogen, compressed
node
   Bouchard
   gouty
   Haygarth
   Heberden
   Meynet
   Schmorl
nodular fasciitis
nodule, rheumatoid
Noiles fully constrained tricompartmental knee prosthesis
NoLok screw
nonbeveled
nonfenestrated stem
nonhinged linked prosthesis

nonicteric sclerae
nonoperative orthopedic management: traction, weights, bed rest
nonsteroidal anti-inflammatory drug (NSAID)
nonsuppurative osteomyelitis
nontender
nonunion
  elephant foot
  horse-hoof
  oligotrophic
  torsion wedge
nonunion of fracture site
nonweightbearing (NWB) brace
normal
  cosmetically and functionally
  upper limits of
Normalize hip prosthesis
Norton ball reamer
Norwood tenodesis
notch
  clavicular
  coracoid
  costal
  cotyloid
  intercondylar
  intervertebral
  scapular
  sciatic
  spinoglenoid
  trochlear
notchplasty
Noyes flexion rotation drawer test
NSAID (nonsteroidal anti-inflammatory drug)
nubbin
Nucleotome system for lumbar diskectomy
nucleus pulposus, herniated (HNP)
nudge control on prosthesis
NuKO knee orthosis
numb, numbness
Nurolon suture
Nylok self-locking nail
NYU (New York University) orthosis

# O, o

OAWO (opening abductory wedge osteotomy)
Ober tendon technique
Ober-Barr procedure for brachioradialis transfer
oblique, obliquity
O'Brien classification of radial fracture
obturator internus muscle
obturator
  conical
  core biopsy
occiput
occupation, sedentary
occupational therapy (OT)
odontoid process
O'Donoghue facetectomy
O'Donoghue triad
O'Donoghue, unhappy triad of
ODQ (opponens digiti quinti)
OEC knee immobilizer
OEC popliteal pad
OEC wrist/forearm support
offset, head-stem
Ogden classification of epiphyseal fracture
Oh hip prosthesis
ointment
Olds pin
olecranon fossa
olisthetic vertebra, wedging of
olisthy
olive
Ollier disease; rake retractor
Omega compression hip screw system
Omer-Capen technique
Omnipaque contrast media
onlay cancellous iliac graft
onycho-osteodysplasia
onychocryptosis (ingrown nail)
Op-Site dressing
open reduction, internal fixation (ORIF)

opening wedge manipulation and reapplication of plaster
operation (see also *amputation*)
Abbott-Fischer-Lucas hip arthrodesis
Abbott-Gill osteotomy
Abbott-Lucas shoulder abduction osteotomy
ablative surgery
Adams arthrodesis
Adams hip adduction osteotomy
Adkins spinal fusion
Akin phalangeal osteotomy
Albee spinal fusion
Allan open reduction of calcaneal fracture
AMBI fixation
Amspacher-Messenbaugh technique
Amstutz-Wilson osteotomy
Anderson-Fowler procedure
Anderson-Hutchins technique
Andrews iliotibial band reconstruction
AO group shoulder arthrodesis
APR cement fixation
Arafiles elbow arthrodesis
Armistead ulnar lengthening
Ashworth hand arthroplasty
ASIF screw fixation technique
Atasoy V-Y technique
atlanto-occipital fusion
Aufranc cup arthroplasty
Austin Moore arthroplasty
Avila technique
avulsion technique
Axer-Clark procedure
Axer varus derotational osteotomy
Baciu-Filibiu dowel ankle arthrodesis
Badgley iliac wing resection
Bailey-Badgley cervical spine fusion
Bailey-Dubow osteotomy
Baker patellar advancement
Baker translocation
Baker-Hill osteotomy

operation *(cont.)*
Balacescu-Golden technique
Bandi technique
Bankart shoulder repair
Bankart-Putti-Platt
Banks-Laufman technique
Barr open reduction and internal fixation
Barr-Record arthrodesis
Barr tendon transfer
Barr tibial fracture fixation
Barrasso-Wile-Gage arthrodesis
Barsky technique
Bartlett nail fold
Batchelor-Brown arthrodesis
Batch-Spittler-McFaddin technique
Bateman hemiarthroplasty
Bateman modification of Mayer transfer
Bauer-Tondra-Trusler
Baumgard-Schwartz tennis elbow technique
Beall-Webel-Bailey technique
Bechtol arthroplasty
Beckenbaugh technique
Becton technique
Bell-Tawse open reduction technique
Bellemore-Barrett-Middleton-Scougall-Whiteway technique
Berman-Gartland metatarsal osteotomy
B.H. Moore procedure
Bickel-Moe procedure
Bircher-Weber technique
Black-Bröstrom staple technique
Blair-Morris-Dunn-Hand ankle arthrodesis
Bleck recession technique
Bloom-Raney modification
Blount displacement osteotomy
Blount tracing technique
Blundell-Jones technique
Bohlman cervical fusion technique
Bonfiglio modification
Bora technique
Borggreve limb rotation

operation (cont.)
Bose nail fold excision
Bosworth bone peg insertion
Bosworth spinal fusion
Boyd-Anderson technique
Boyd-Bosworth procedure
Boyd-McLeod tennis elbow technique
Boyd-Sisk posterior capsulorrhaphy
Boyes brachioradialis transfer technique
Brackett-Osgood-Putti-Abbott
Brady-Jewett technique
Brain arthroplasty
Brand tendon transfer technique
Brannon-Wickstrom technique
Brantigan-Voshell procedure
Braun procedure
Brett-Campbell tibial osteotomy
Bristow-Helfet procedure
Bristow-May procedure
Brittain arthrodesis
Brookes-Jones tendon transfer
Brooks-Jenkins atlantoaxial fusion
Brooks-Seddon transfer technique
Brown knee joint reconstruction
Bruser technique
Bryan arthroplasty
Bryan-Morrey technique
Buck-Gramcko technique
Bugg-Boyd technique
Buncke technique
Bunnell tendon transfer technique
Burgess technique
Burkhalter transfer technique
Burrows technique
Butler fifth toe
Calandriello procedure
Calandruccio fixation
calcaneonavicular bar resection
calcaneotibial fusion
Caldwell-Coleman flatfoot technique
Caldwell-Durham tendon technique
Callahan fusion technique
Camitz technique
Campbell-Akbarnia arthrodesis

operation (cont.)
Campbell-Goldthwait procedure
Canale osteotomy
capitellocondylar arthroplasty
Carceau-Brahms ankle arthrodesis
Carnesale technique
Carrell fibular substitution
Castle procedure
Cave-Rowe shoulder dislocation
Chandler arthrodesis
Chandler hip fusion
Chapchal knee arthrodesis
Charcot hip arthrodesis
Charnley compression-type knee fusion
Charnley-Houston arthrodesis
Chaves-Rapp muscle transfer
chemonucleolysis
Chiari innominate osteotomy
Childress ankle fixation technique
Cho cruciate ligament reconstruction
Chrisman-Snook ankle technique
Chuinard-Peterson ankle arthrodesis
Clancy ligament technique
Clark transfer technique
Clayton-Fowler technique
Cleveland-Bosworth-Thompson
closed manipulative
Cloward back fusion
Cloward cervical arthrodesis
Cobb scoliosis measuring technique
Codivilla tendon lengthening
Cole tendon fixation
Coleman flatfoot technique
Collis broken femoral stem technique
Colonna trochanteric arthroplasty
Coltart fracture technique
Compere-Thompson arthrodesis
Coonrad total elbow arthroplasty
Coonse-Adams technique
costotransversectomy technique
Couch-Derosa-Throop transfer
Coventry vagus osteotomy
Cozen-Brockway technique
Cracchiolo forefoot arthroplasty

"Derek" = Darrach

operation (cont.)
Crawford-Adams cup arthroplasty
Crego tendon transfer technique
Cubbins arthroplasty
Curtin plantar fibromatosis excision
Curtis-Fisher knee technique
Curtis PIP joint capsulotomy
Darrach-McLaughlin technique
Das Gupta procedure
d'Aubigne femoral reconstruction
Davey-Rorabeck-Fowler technique
Davis drainage technique
De Andrade-MacNab occipito-cervical arthrodesis
Debeyre-Patte-Elmelik rotator cuff decompression technique
degloving procedure
Dennyson-Fulford subtalar arthrodesis
Dewar-Barrington arthroplasty
Dewar-Harris shoulder technique
Deyerle femoral fracture technique
Diamond-Gould syndactyly
Dias-Giegerich fracture technique
Dickinson-Coutts-Woodward-Handler osteotomy
Dickson transplant technique
Dimon-Hughston fracture fixation
Doll trochanteric reattachment
Dorrance procedure
doweling spondylolisthesis
Drez modification of Eriksson technique
Drummond wire technique
Dunn-Brittain foot stabilization
Dunn-Hess trochanteric osteotomy
Durham flatfoot
duToit-Roux arthroplasty
duToit-Roux staple capsulorrhaphy
DuVries reconstruction technique
Dwyer clawfoot
Eaton arthroplasty
Eaton-Littler technique
Eaton-Malerich fracture-dislocation
Eberle contracture release
Ecker-Lotke-Glazer tendon reconstruction

operation (cont.)
Eden-Hybbinette arthroplasty
Eden-Lange procedure
Edward procedure
Eftekhar broken femoral stem technique
Eggers tendon transfer technique
Elizabethtown osteotomy
Ellis Jones peroneal tendon
Ellison lateral knee reconstruction
Elmslie-Trillat transplant
Emmon osteotomy
Ender fracture technique
Enneking knee arthrodesis
Eppright dial osteotomy
Erickson-Leider-Brown technique
Eriksson reconstruction
Essex-Lopresti axial fixation
Essex-Lopresti open reduction
Evans osteotomy
Ewald-Walker knee arthroplasty
Eyler flexorplasty
Fahey technique
Fairbanks technique with Sever modification
Farmer
Ferciot-Thomson excision
Ferguson-Thompson-King two-stage osteotomy
Ferkel torticollis
Fernandez osteotomy
Ficat procedure
Fish cuneiform osteotomy
five-one reconstruction
Flynn
forage
Forbes modification of Phemister graft
Fowler procedure
four-bar external fixation
Fowler tendon transfer
Fowles dislocation
Fox-Blazina procedure
free body fusion technique
French supracondylar fracture
Fried-Hendel tendon

operation *(cont.)*
Froimson procedure
Furnas-Haq-Somers technique
Gaenslen technique
Galeazzi patellar
Gallie subtalar fusion
Gant osteotomy
Garceau-Brahms arthrodesis
Gardner
Gartland procedure
Getty decompression technique
Ghormley arthrodesis
Giannestras metatarsal oblique osteotomy
Gibson-Piggott osteotomy
Gilbert-Tamai-Weiland technique
Gill-Manning-White spondylolisthesis
Gill-Stein arthrodesis
Gillies-Millard cocked-hat technique
Girdlestone-Taylor procedure
Glynn-Neibauer technique
Goldner-Clippinger technique
Goldstein spinal fusion
Goldthwait-Hauser procedure
Gordon-Broström technique
Gordon-Taylor technique
Gouffon fixation
Green-Banks technique
Greenfield osteotomy
Greulich-Pyle technique
Grice-Green arthrodesis
Gristina-Webb shoulder arthroplasty
Grosse-Kempf tibial technique
Groves-Goldner technique
Guller resection
Guttmann arthrodesis
Guyon tunnel release
Haddad-Riordan arthrodesis
Hall facet fusion
hanging toe
Harmon transfer technique
Harrington rod fixation
Harrington total hip arthroplasty
Harris-Beath arthrodesis
Harris-Smith cervical fusion

operation *(cont.)*
Hass procedure
Hassmann-Brunn-Neer elbow technique
Hauser patellar technique
hemiarthroplasty
Henderson arthrodesis
Henry-Geist spinal fusion
Hey-Groves-Kirk technique
Heyman-Herndon-Strong technique
Hibbs-Jones spinal fusion
Hill-Nahai-Vasconez-Mathes technique
His-Haas procedure
Hitchcock tendon technique
Hohmann procedure
Hoke arthrodesis
Hoppenfeld-Deboer technique
Horwitz-Adams ankle fusion
Houghton-Akroyd technique
Hovnanian transfer technique
Howard technique
Howorth procedure
Hughston-Degenhardt reconstruction
Hughston-Hauser procedure
Hughston-Jacobson technique
Hungerford-Krackow-Kenna knee arthroplasty
Huntington tibial technique
I-beam hip
ICLH double cup arthroplasty
Ilizarov leg lengthening technique
implant
Inclan-Ober procedure
Inglis-Cooper technique
Inglis-Ranawat-Straub technique
Ingram bony bridge resection
Insall-Burstein-Freeman knee arthroplasty
interpositional elbow arthroplasty
intra-articular knee fusion
Jaffe procedure
Jansey technique
Japas osteotomy
Jeffery technique

operation *(cont.)*
John C. Wilson arthrodesis
Johnson pelvic fracture technique
Johnson-Spiegl hallux varus correction
Jones-Brackett technique
J.R. Moore procedure
Kapel elbow dislocation technique
Kaplan technique
Karakousis-Vezeridis procedure
Kashiwagi technique
Kate procedure
Kates-Kessel-Kay technique
Kaufer tendon technique
Kelikian-Clayton-Loseff technique
Kelikian-McFarland procedure
Kelikian-Riashi-Gleason technique
Keller resection arthroplasty
Kellogg-Speed fusion technique
Kendrick-Sharma-Hassler-Herndon
Kennedy ligament technique
Kessel-Bonney extension osteotomy
Kessler technique
Key arthrodesis
Key intra-articular knee arthrodesis
keyhole tenodesis
Kickaldy-Willis arthrodesis
Kidner foot procedure
King-Richards dislocation technique
King-Steelquist technique
Klein technique
Klisic-Jankovic technique
Knobby-Clark procedure
Kocher-McFarland hip arthroplasty
Koutsogiannis-Fowler-Anderson osteotomy
Kramer-Craig-Noel osteotomy
Krempen-Silver-Sotelo nonunion
Kronner external fixation
Krukenberg
Kumar spica cast technique
Kumar-Cowell-Ramsey technique
Lamb muscle transfer
Lambrinudi technique
Lange procedure
Langenskiöld bony bridge resection

operation *(cont.)*
Lapidus hammer toe technique
Larmon forefoot procedure
Larson ligament reconstruction
Leach-Igou step-cut medial osteotomy
Lehman
Lenart-Kullman technique
L'Episcopo-Zachary technique
Lewis-Chekofsky resection
Lichtman technique
Liebolt radioulnar technique
limb-sparing
Lindeman procedure
Lindholm technique
Lipscomb modified McKeever arthrodesis
Littler-Cooley technique
Lloyd-Roberts fracture technique
Localio procedure
Loose procedure
Lorenz procedure
Losee modification of MacIntosh
Lucas-Murray knee arthrodesis
Luque rod fixation
MacAusland procedure
MacCarthy procedure
MacEwen-Shands osteotomy
MacIntosh over-the-top repair
MacIntosh tenodesis
MacNab
Magilligan measuring technique
Magnuson-Stack shoulder arthrotomy
Majestro-Ruda-Frost tendon
Malawer excision technique
Mankin technique
Manktelow transfer procedure
Mann modified McKeever arthrodesis
Mann-DuVries arthroplasty
Manske technique
Maquet technique
Marcus-Balourdas-Heiple ankle fusion
Marks-Bayne thumb duplication

operation *(cont.)*
  Marshall ligament repair
  Martin osteotomy
  Matchett-Brown hip arthroplasty
  Matti-Russe technique
  Mauck procedure
  Mayo total elbow arthroplasty
  Mazet technique
  McCarroll-Baker procedure
  McConnell technique
  McElfresh-Dobyns-O'Brien
  McFarland-Osborne technique
  McKeever medullary clavicle fixation
  McKeever-Buck elbow technique
  McLaughlin-Hay technique
  McReynolds open reduction
  Memford-Gurd arthroplasty
  Mensor-Scheck technique
  Meyerding-Van Demark technique
  Milch cuff resection
  Milch elbow technique
  Millender-Nalebuff wrist arthrodesis
  Miller flatfoot
  Miller-Galante arthroplasty
  Millesi modified technique
  Mital elbow release technique
  Mitchell osteotomy
  Mizuno technique
  Moberg-Gedda open reduction
  modified Hoke-Miller flatfoot procedure
  modified mold and surface replacement arthroplasty
  Moe scoliosis technique
  monofilament wire fixation
  monospherical shoulder arthroplasty
  Monticelli-Spinelli distraction
  Moore technique
  Morgan-Casscells meniscus suturing
  Morrey-Bryan elbow arthroplasty
  Morrison technique
  Mubarak-Hargens decompression
  Mueller (Müller) hip arthroplasty
  Mumford-Gurd acromioclavicular
  Nalebuff-Millender technique

operation *(cont.)*
  Naughton-Dunn triple arthrodesis
  Neer unconstrained shoulder arthroplasty
  neural arch resection
  Neviaser-Wilson-Gardner technique
  New England Baptist hip arthroplasty
  Nicholas five-in-one reconstruction
  Nicoll fracture
  Niebauer-King technique
  Nirschl
  Ober-Barr transfer technique
  O'Brien pelvic halo
  O'Donoghue ACL reconstruction
  Ollier technique
  Omer-Capen technique
  ORIF (open reduction, internal fixation)
  Osborne-Cotterill elbow dislocation
  Osgood rotational osteotomy
  Ostrup technique
  Pack technique
  Palmer-Widen shoulder technique
  pan-talar arthrodesis
  pants-over-vest technique
  Papineau technique
  parapatellar arthrotomy
  patellar tendon transfer (PTT)
  Paterson technique
  Paulos ligament technique
  Pauwels proximal osteotomy
  Pauwels Y osteotomy
  Peacock transposing technique
  Pemberton pericapsular osteotomy
  percutaneous pin insertion
  Perry-Nickel technique
  Perry-O'Brien-Hodgson technique
  Perry-Robinson cervical technique
  Pheasant elbow technique
  Phemister onlay bone graft
  Platou osteotomy
  Post shoulder arthroplasty
  Pott eversion osteotomy
  Putti knee arthrodesis
  Putti-Platt arthroplasty

operation *(cont.)*
Radley-Liebig-Brown resection
reefing
Reichenheim-King procedure
resurfacing
Reverdin osteotomy
reverse Mauck procedure
Ridlon procedure
Robinnson-Chung-Farahvar morcellation
Robinson-Riley cervical arthrodesis
Robinson-Southwick fusion
Rockwood-Green technique
Rogers cervical fusion technique
Root-Siegal osteotomy
Roux-duToit staple capsulorrhaphy
Roux-Goldthwait procedure
Rowe-Zarins shoulder immobilization
Ruiz-Mora procedure
Russe technique
Ryerson triple arthrodesis
Sage-Clark technique
Saha transfer technique
Salter pelvic osteotomy
Samilson osteotomy
Sarmiento trochanteric fracture technique
Scaglietti closed reduction technique
Schaberg-Harper-Allen technique
Schanz angulation osteotomy
Schauwecker patellar wiring
Schlein elbow arthroplasty
Schneider hip arthrodesis
Schnute wedge resection technique
Schrock procedure
Scott glenoplasty
Scuderi technique
Seddon modification
Sell-Frank-Johnson extensor shift
Sharrard transfer technique
shelf
Sherk-Probst technique
shish kebab technique
Shriver-Johnson arthrodesis
Siffert-Forster-Nachamie arthrodesis

operation *(cont.)*
Siffert-Storen intraepiphyseal osteotomy
Silfverskiöld technique
Silver bunionectomy
Simmonds-Menelaus metatarsal osteotomy
Simmons cervical spine fusion
Skoog technique
Slocum fusion technique
Smith-Petersen cup arthroplasty
Smith-Petersen sacroiliac joint fusion
Smith-Robinson cervical fusion
Sofield femoral deficiency technique
Somerville technique
Southwick slide procedure
Speed arthroplasty
Speed-Boyd radial-ulnar technique
Spier elbow arthrodesis
Spira procedure
Spittler procedure
Sponsel oblique osteotomy
Stack shoulder procedure
Staheli shelf procedure
Stamm procedure
Stanisavljevic technique
Stanmore shoulder arthroplasty
Staples elbow arthrodesis
Staples-Black-Broström ligament repair
Stark-Moore-Ashworth-Boyes technique
Steel triple innominate osteotomy
Steindler flexorplasty
Stewart-Harley ankle arthrodesis
Stiles-Bunnell transfer technique
Strayer tendon technique
Sugioka transtrochanteric osteotomy
surface replacement
Sutherland-Greenfield osteotomy
Swanson Convex condylar arthroplasty
Swanson silicone wrist arthroplasty
symmetric vertebral fusion
Tachdjian hamstring lengthening
Taylor-Daniel-Weiland technique

operation *(cont.)*
tension band fixation
terminal Syme procedure
Teuffer technique
Thomas-Thompson-Straub transfer
Thompson telescoping V osteotomy
Thompson-Henry technique
tibiotalar fusion
Tikhoff-Linberg procedure
Tohen tendon technique
Torg knee reconstruction
Torgerson-Leach modified technique
total articular resurfacing arthroplasty (TARA)
total hip arthroplasty
total knee arthroplasty
transmalleolar ankle arthrodesis
Trethowan-Stamm-Simmonds, Menelaus-Haddad triangulation
triaxial total elbow arthroplasty
Trillat procedure
triple arthrodesis
Trumble arthrodesis
Turco clubfoot release
two-sleeve technique
two-stage hip fusion
Uematsu arthrodesis
Vastamäki technique
vastus medialis advancement
Veleanu-Rosianu-Ionescu technique
Verdan technique
Vidal-Ardrey fracture technique
Vitallium cup arthroplasty
Volz-Turner reattachment
Vulpius-Compere tendon technique
Wadsworth technique
Wagner open reduction technique
Wagoner cervical technique
Warner-Farber ankle fixation
Watkins fusion technique
Watson-Cheyne technique
Watson-Jones arthrodesis
Weaver-Dunn acromioclavicular
Weber-Brunner-Freuler-Boitzy
Weber-Vasey traction-absorption
West and Soto-Hall patella

operation *(cont.)*
White arthrodesis
Whitecloud-LaRocca arthrodesis
Whitesides-Kelly cervical technique
Whitman osteotomy
Williams-Haddad technique
Wilson-Jacobs tibial fixation
Wilson-Johansson-Barrington arthrodesis
Wilson-McKeever arthroplasty
Wiltse ankle osteotomy
Winograd (ingrown nail) technique
Winter spondylolisthesis
Wirth-Jager tendon technique
Woodward technique
Yoke transposition procedure
Yount procedure
Zancolli rerouting technique
Zaricznyj ligament technique
Zarins-Rowe ligament technique
Zazepen-Gamidov technique
Zeier transfer technique
Zickel nail fixation
Zickel subtrochanteric fracture
Oppenheim brace; disease; sign
Oppenheimer spring wire splint
opposition
Opraflex incise drape
Optifix prosthesis
O'Rahilly classification of limb deficiency
Oregon Poly II ankle prosthesis
Oretorp arthroscopy knife
organomegaly
oriented x 3 (to time, place, person)
ORIF (open reduction, internal fixation)
origin, muscle
Oris pin
Orr-Buck traction
Orthawear antiembolism stocking
Ortho-Cel padding
Ortho-Foam protector
Ortho-Trac bandage
Ortho-Vent bandage; traction
Orthochrome implant metal

Orthofix device
Orthofix external fixator
OrthoGen implantable stimulator for
 nonunion of fracture
Ortholav jet lavage
Ortholoc implant metal
orthopedic bed (see *bed*)
orthopedic hardware
orthopedist (also *orthopaedist*)
orthopod
orthosis (see also *brace; splint*)
 A-frame
 abduction hip
 airplane splint
 ankle-foot
 Atlanta brace
 bail-lock knee joint
 Boston brace thoracolumbosacral
 C-bar
 cable twister
 cervical
 cervicothoracolumbosacral (CTLSO)
 chairback
 cock-up splint
 Denis Browne bar foot
 dial lock
 elastic knee cage
 elastic twister
 elbow-wrist-hand (EWHO)
 figure-of-8 thoracic
 Fillauer bar foot
 flexion-extension control cervical
 floor-reaction ankle-foot
 four-poster cervical
 Frejka pillow
 gator plastic
 halo extension; traction
 heat-molded petroplastic ankle-foot
 hip-knee-ankle-foot (HKAFO)
 Ilfield splint
 Jewett thoracolumbosacral
 Klenzak
 knee-ankle-foot (KAFO)
 Knight-Taylor thoracolumbosacral
 Legg-Perthes disease
 Lenox Hill knee

orthosis *(cont.)*
 Lerman multiligamentous knee
  control
 long leg
 long opponens
 LSU reciprocation-gait
 Milwaukee cervicothoracolumbosacral
 molded
 Newington
 NuKO knee
 parapodium
 Phelps
 Plastizote collar cervical
 plastic floor reaction ankle-foot
 PTB (patellar tendon bearing)
  ankle-foot
 PTB plastic
 rib belt
 safety pin
 Scottish Rite hip
 semirigid
 short opponens
 shoulder-elbow-wrist-hand
  (SEWHO)
 soft collar cervical
 SOMI (skull-occiput-mandibular
  immobilization)
 spring-loaded lock
 spring wire ankle-foot
 standing frame
 Swedish knee cage
 Taylor thoracolumbosacral
 thermoplastic ankle-foot
 Thomas collar cervical
 thoracolumbosacral (TLSO)
 Toronto
 total contact (TCO)
 trilateral knee-ankle-foot
 two-poster cervical
 UCB (University of California,
  Berkeley) foot
 underarm
 Von Rosen splint hip
 Williams
 wrist-driven flexor hinge

os acromiale
os peroneum

orthosis overlapped uprights
orthotist
orthotome resector
Ortolani maneuver; sign
os intermetatarseum
os tibiale externum
os trigonum
Osborne-Cotterill elbow technique
oscillating saw (see *saw*)
Osgood modified technique
Osgood-Schlatter disease
osseous outgrowth
ossicle
ossification
   enchondral
   endochondral
   heterotopic
ossimeter
Ossotome bur
ostealgia
ostectomy, fibular
osteitis deformans
osteitis fibrosa cystica
osteitis fragilitans
osteitis ossificans
osteitis pubis
osteitis, sclerosing nonsuppurative
ostempyesis
Osteo-Stim implantable bone growth
   stimulator
osteoaneurysm
osteoarthritis
osteoarthropathy
osteoarthrosis
osteoblastic bone regeneration
osteoblastoma
osteocachexia
osteoclast
osteocartilaginous metaplasia
osteochondral graft
osteochondritis deformans juvenilis
osteochondritis dissecans
osteochondritis, epiphyseal
osteochondritis ischiopubica
osteochondritis juvenilis

osteochondritis necroticans
osteochondrofibroma
osteochondrolysis
osteochondroma, epiphyseal
osteochondromatosis, synovial
osteochondropathy
osteochondrophyte
osteochondrosarcoma
osteochondrosis deformans tibiae
osteochondrosis dissecans
osteoclasis, Blount technique for
osteoclast
osteoclastoma
osteocope
osteocystoma
osteocyte
osteodiastasis
osteodynia
osteodystrophy
   azotemic
   renal
osteoenchondroma
osteofibrochondrosarcoma
osteofibromatosis
OsteoGen implantable stimulator for
   nonunion of fracture
osteogenesis imperfecta
osteogenic sarcoma (see *sarcoma*)
osteohalisteresis
osteoid osteoma
osteolipochondroma
osteolipoma
osteolysis
osteoma, osteoid
osteomalacia
osteomatosis
osteomized
osteomyelitic sinus
osteomyelitis
   acute hematogenous
   blastomycotic
   Garre sclerosing
   iatrogenic
   nonsuppurative
   post-traumatic chronic

osteomyelodysplasia
osteonal bone
osteonecrosis, dysbaric
osteoneuralgia
Osteonics hip prosthesis
osteopathia striata
osteopathy
osteopenia
osteoperiosteal graft
osteoperiostitis
osteopetrosis
osteophytes
  bridging
  fringe of
  marginal
osteophytosis
osteoplastica
osteopoikilosis
osteoporosis, osteoporotic
osteopsathyrosis idiopathica
osteoradionecrosis
osteosarcoma
  parosteal
  periosteal
  telangiectatic
osteosclerosis fragilis
osteosis
osteospongioma
Osteo-Stim bone stimulator,
  battery-pack
Osteo-Stim, Zimmer
osteosynovitis
osteosynthesis
osteotabes
osteotelangiectasia
osteothrombophlebitis
osteothrombosis
osteotome
  Albee
  Army
  bayonet
  Blount
  Bowen
  box
  Campbell
  Carroll-Legg

osteotome *(cont.)*
  Carroll-Smith-Petersen
  Cavin
  Cherry
  Clayton
  Cloward
  Cobb
  Compere
  Cottle
  Crane
  curved
  grooving
  guarded
  Hibbs curved; straight
  Hoke
  Joseph
  Meyerding curved; straight
  rotary
  Simmons
  Smith-Petersen curved; straight
  straight
  thin
  unguarded
  Weck
osteotomize
osteotomy (see *operation)*
  abduction (hip)
  adduction (hip)
  ball-and-socket
  basilar
  bifurcation
  biplane trochanteric
  calcaneal
  chevron
  closed wedge
  closing abductory wedge (CAWO)
  closing wedge
  crescentic
  cuneiform
  cup-and-ball
  delayed femoral
  derotational
  dial pelvic
  dome-shaped
  double
  extension

osteotomy *(cont.)*
  flexion
  geometric extension
  innominate
  intertrochanteric
  intracapsular
  lateral closing wedge
  malleolar
  medial displacement
  medial opening wedge
  metatarsal neck
  oblique, with derotation
  open wedge
  opening abductory wedge (OAWO)
  opening wedge
  peg-in-hole
  Sofield
  supracondylar varus
  supramalleolar
  tarsal wedge
  through-and-through V-shaped horizontal
  tibial
  trapezoidal
  triplane
  valgus
  varus derotational
  wedge-shaped
osteotomy-osteoclasis, Moore
Ostrup technique
OT (occupational therapy)
Otto pelvis dislocation
outgrowth, osseous patellae
Outerbridge scale for joint or articular surface damage in chondromalacia patellae
Overdyke hip prosthesis
overextension
overgrowth
overlap, overlapped
overlapped uprights in orthosis
overpull
overriding
oversewn
Overton dowel graft
Owens silk

Owestry staple
oxygen, hyperbaric

# P, p

Pack technique
pack
  hot
  vaginal
packing, Adaptic
pad, pads
  ABD (abdominal)
  abdominal lap
  Arthropor
  buttock
  digital
  fat
  Hapad medial arch
  heel
  horseshoe-shaped felt
  knee-control orthosis
  knuckle
  lamb's wool
  Mik
  Mikulicz
  navicular shoe
  OEC popliteal
  patellar orthosis
  pubic
  Redigrip knee
  reticulated polyurethane
  scaphoid shoe
  shoe heel
  spur
pad/protector, Decubinex
padding
  contoured felt
  cotton cast
  felt
  Ortho-Cel

Paget associated osteogenic sarcoma
pagetoid bone
pain
   contralateral
   dull aching
   joint line
   lancinating
   phantom
   radicular
   referred
pain at rest
pain with weightbearing
Pais fracture
Palacos cement
palindromic rheumatism
palmar crease
palmaris longus tendon
Palmer-Widen shoulder technique
palpation
palsy
   backpack
   Erb-Duchenne
   handlebar
   Klumpke
   median nerve
   peroneal
   radial nerve
   sciatic
   tardy median nerve
   tardy ulnar nerve
   ulnar nerve
Panner disease
pannus of synovium
pan-talar arthrodesis
Pantopaque
panty/girdle, Cadenza
paper, tracing
Papineau grafting; technique
PAR (postanesthesia recovery)
para-articular calcification
parallel
paralysis
   Chaves-Rapp
   Dewar-Harris
   Dickson
   familial periodic

paralysis *(cont.)*
   Haas
   Henry
   Vastamäki
   Volkmann ischemic
   Whitman
paralysis agitans
paramedian sagittal plane
parapatellar plica
paraplegia, paraplegic
parasagittal scar
paraspinal musculature
parasternal heave
paratenon
paravertebral musculature
paresis
paresthesias, intermittent
Parham-Martin fracture apparatus
parietal pleura
Parkinson disease
Parona space
paronychia
parosteal osteogenic sarcoma
Parrish-Mann hammertoe technique
pars interarticularis
particles of bone
particulate debris
passer
   Brand tendon
   Bunnell tendon
   suture
   tendon
paste, Unna
Patel medial meniscectomy
patella
   bipartite
   dislocated
   high-riding
   minima
   subluxing
   undersurface of
patella alta
patella minima
patellapexy
patellar advancement, Baker
patellar button

patellar contour, Wiberg type II
patellar dislocation
patellar edge
patellar fat pad
patellar groove
patellar instability
patellar jerk
patellar orthosis pad
patellar tendon bearing (PTB) cast
patellar tracking
patellectomy, Soto-Hall
patellofemoral crepitation
patelloquadriceps tendon
Paterson procedure
pathognomonic sign
Patrick test
pattern
   DISI collapse
   storiform
   gait
patty
   cement
   cottonoid
Paulos ligament technique
Pauwels Y osteotomy
Pavlik bandage; harness; sling; splint
Payr sign
PB (paraffin bath)
PCA (porous-coated anatomic) prosthesis
PCL (posterior cruciate ligament)
Peabody splint
Peacock transposing technique
Pearson attachment to Thomas splint
Pease-Thomson traction
pectus carinatum
pectus excavatum
pedicle, pedicled
pedicle, vascular
pedorthotist
pedunculated
peg
   bone
      fixation
pegging

Pellegrini-Stieda disease
pelvic brim
pelvic traction
pelvis, Otto
Pemberton pericapsular osteotomy
PEMF (pulsating electromagnetic field)
pen, skin-marking
pencil
   electrosurgical
   skin
penciling of ribs on x-ray
Penfield dissector; elevator
Penrose drain
per primam healing
perception, constant-touch
periarticular fibrositis
pericyte, Zimmerman
perimysiitis
perimysium
perineural
perineurial neurorrhaphy
periosteal elevator (see *elevator*)
periosteotome
   Alexander-Farabeuf
   Ballender
   Brown
periosteotomy
periosteum, periosteal
periostitis
peripheral pulses symmetrical and intact
Perkins traction; line
peroneal nerve
peroneus brevis
peroneus longus
peroxide flush
perpendicular
Perry-Nickel technique
Perry-O'Brien-Hodgson technique
Perry-Robinson cervical technique
Perthes disease
pes anserinus
pes cavus
pes equinus
pes plantigrade planus

*Handwritten annotations at top:*
*pilon fracture also to Kary*
*pylon fracture also possible*
*pillion fracture also possible*

pes planus, rigid
petechia, petechiae
Peterson traction
Petit triangle
Petrie spica cast
Peyronie disease
PFFD (proximal focal femoral deficiency)
PGP nail
phalanx, waist of the
Phalen maneuver; position; test
phantom sensation
Pheasant elbow technique
Phelps brace; orthosis; scapulectomy
Phemister onlay bone graft technique
Phemister-Bonfiglio technique
phenol matricectomy
phenolization
Philadelphia collar cervical support
Philadelphia Plastizote cervical brace
Phillips head screwdriver
phocomelia
Phoenix hip prosthesis
photon densitometry
photoplethysmography
physical therapy (PT)
physiotherapy
pi, locating
pickups
piece, chin-occiput
piecemeal
Piedmont fracture
Pierrot-Murphy tendon technique
pillow
   abduction
   Bio-Gel decubitus
   Carter elevation
   cervical
   elevate on
   Frejka
   PRN
pilonidal dimple
pin (see also *pinning*)
   alignment
   Austin Moore
   ball guide

pin *(cont.)*
   ball-point guide
   ball-tip guide
   beaded reamer guide
   Beath
   Bilos
   Böhler
   Bohlman
   calcaneal
   calibrated
   Canakis
   Charnley
   clavicle
   collapsible
   Compere threaded
   Compton clavicle
   Conley
   Crego-McCarroll
   Davis
   Day
   DePuy
   Deyerle II
   drill
   Ender
   Fahey-Compere
   femoral guide
   Fischer transfixing
   fixation
   Gouffon hip
   guide
   Hagie hip
   half
   halo
   Hansen-Street
   Hare
   Hatcher
   Haynes
   intramedullary
   Jones compression
   Knowles
   Küntscher
   locating
   Lottes
   marble bone
   McBride
   Modny

pin *(cont.)*
   Moore
   Olds
   Oris
   percutaneous
   Pitcock
   precurved ball-tipped guide
   Pritchard Mark II
   Rhinelander
   Riordan
   Roger Anderson
   Rush
   Schanz
   Schneider
   Schweitzer
   self-broaching
   Serrato forearm
   Shriner
   Smith-Petersen
   smooth Steinmann
   socket
   Stader
   Steinmann, with ball-bearing
   Street medullary
   strut-type
   threaded
   threaded Steinmann
   traction
   transarticular
   transfixing
   Turner
   Varney
   Venable-Stuck
   Vom Saal
   wrench
   Zimmer
pin chuck, Steinmann pin with
pin fixation (see *operation)*
pinch power, thumb
pinch, key
pinning (see also *pin)*
   closed
   in situ
   Knowles
   open
   percutaneous

pinning *(cont.)*
   Sofield
   Wagner closed
pinprick sensation
Piotrowski sign
PIP (proximal interphalangeal) joint
PIPJ (proximal interphalangeal joint)
Pipkin classification of femoral
   fracture
Pirogoff amputation
Pischel micropin
piston, cannulated expulsion
piston sign (on x-ray)
pistoning
Pitcock nail; pin
Pittsburgh pelvic frame
pivot-shift test; sign
plafond, tibial
plane
   anatomic
   axial
   coronal
   fascial
   flexion-extension
   frontal
   Hensen
   Hodge
   horizontal
   internervous
   intertubercular
   Ludwig
   median sagittal
   mesiodistal
   midsagittal
   paramedian sagittal
   pelvic
   sagittal
   spinous
   sternoxiphoid
   subcostal
   suprasternal
   thoracic
   transverse
   varus-valgus
   vertical
plantar axial view

plantar flexion-inversion deformity
plantar response
plantar flexed
plantaris muscle
plantarward
planum
plasmacytoma, extramedullary
plaster of Paris, elastic
plaster-of-Paris cast
plaster toe cap
plaster, Zoroc
plastic, thermolabile
Plastizote cervical collar orthosis
plate
  anchor
  AO condylar blade
  AO contoured T
  AO small fragment
  AOI blade
  ASIF right-angle blade
  Badgley
  Bagby angled compression
  Batchelor
  Blount blade
  bone
  Bosworth spine
  Burns
  buttress
  Calandruccio side
  cap-and-anchor
  cartilaginous growth
  cloverleaf
  coaptation
  cobra-head
  Collison
  compression
  contoured T-plate
  cortical
  DCP (dynamic compression)
  DePuy
  Deyerle
  Driessen hinged
  dual
  Duopress
  dynamic compression (DCP)
  Eggers bone

plate *(cont.)*
  Elliott femoral condyle blade
  epiphyseal
  femoral
  fibrocartilaginous
  five-hole
  fixed-angle blade
  four-hole
  heavy-duty femur
  Gallannaugh
  growth
  Hagie sliding nail
  Hansen-Street
  Harlow
  Harris
  heavy side
  Hicks lugged
  Hoen skull
  Holt nail
  Hubbard
  intertrochanteric
  Jergesen I-beam
  Jergesen tapered
  Jewett nail overlay
  Jones compression
  Kessel
  Laing
  Lane
  Lawson-Thornton
  Letournel
  Lundholm
  Massie
  McBride
  McLaughlin
  Mears sacroiliac
  Meurig Williams
  Milch
  Moe intertrochanteric
  Moore sliding nail
  Moreira
  Müller compression blade
  nail
  Neufeld
  neutralization
  Newman
  Nicoll

| plate | 100 | point |

plate *(cont.)*
  Osborne
  overlay
  peg-base
  plain pattern
  pterygoid
  Pugh
  pylon attachment
  quadrangular positioning plate
  Richards side
  Schweitzer spring
  semitubular
  semitubular compression
  Senn
  serpentine
  Sherman
  Sherman bone
  side
  slide
  slotted femur
  Smith-Petersen
  SMO
  Steffe
  stem base
  subchondral
  Synthes
  T
  T buttress
  T-shaped AO
  tarsal
  Temple University
  Thornton nail
  Townley tibial plateau
  Townsend-Gilfillan
  trial base
  Tupman
  UCP compression
  Uslenghi
  V nail
  V blade
  Venable
  Vitallium
  volar
  Wainwright
  Wenger
  Whitman

plate *(cont.)*
  Wilson
  wing
  Wright
  Y bone
  Zimmer femoral condyle blade
  Zimmer side
  Zimmer Y
  Zuelzer hook
plateau, tibial
Platou osteotomy
platyspondylosis
pledget of gauze
pledget, Betadine-soaked
pleomorphic
plethysmography
  digital
  impedance
plexus, brachial
plica, plicae
  medial
  parapatellar
  suprapatellar
  synovial
plication
  disk
  soft tissue
plicectomy
pliers, needle-nose
plug
  bone
  Buck
  cement
PMI-6A1-4V implant metal
PMMA (antibiotic-impregnated polymethyl methacrylate)
pneumatic tourniquet cuff
pneumoarthrogram
podiatry, podiatrist
point
  bleeding
  Crowe pilot
  dorsal
  drill
  end
  Erb

point *(cont.)*
  glenoid
  Krackow
  Pauly
  pressure
  trigger
  twist drill
point tenderness
POL (posterior oblique ligament)
Poland classification of epiphyseal fracture
pollicization, Buck-Gramcko
polyacetal resin
polyarteritis nodosa
polyarthritis
polyarthropathy
Polycentric and Wide-Track knee system
polydactyly
Polydek suture
Poly-Dial prosthesis
polyethylene proximal brims in quadrilateral contour
polymer
  cold-curing
  self-curing
polymerized
polymethyl methacrylate (PMMA)
polymyositis
polypropylene insert
polytrauma
polyurethane cast
polyvinylalcohol splinting material
Pond adjustable splint
Ponseti splint
POP bandage (plaster of Paris)
pop, popping
popliteal recess
Porocoat AML noncemented prosthesis
Porometal noncemented femoral prosthesis
poroplastic splint
portable C-arm image intensifier fluoroscopy

portal
  arthroscopic entry
  patellar
  superolateral
  superomedial
  Swedish
Porter-Richardson-Vainio technique
porthole
portion
  accessory
  cord
Porzett splint
Posey belt
position
  barber chair
  bayonet fracture
  beach chair
  Bonner
  Brickner
  decubitus
  dorsal
  dorsal lithotomy
  dorsal recumbent
  figure 4
  Fowler
  frogleg
  Gaynor-Hart
  horizontal
  Jones
  jumper's knee
  kneeling
  Kraske
  lateral decubitus
  lithotomy
  lotus
  neutral
  normal anatomic
  Phalen
  prayer
  prone
  rectus
  reverse Trendelenburg
  scissor-leg
  semi-Fowler
  Sims
  spinal fusion

position (cont.)
  supine
  Trendelenburg
position of function, splinted in
positioner
  acetabular cup
  cup
  Montreal hip
  Post total shoulder arthroplasty
post
  Mose tapered prosthetic
  perineal
  thumb
Postalume finger splint
postanesthesia recovery (PAR)
Postel hip status system
posterolateral aspect
postmenopausal
postoperative wound care
postreduction x-ray
posttraumatic chronic osteomyelitis
posture
  decerebrate
  decorticate
Pott eversion osteotomy; splint
pouch, suprapatellar
Poupart inguinal ligament
powder, thrombin
Pratt technique
PREs (progressive resistive exercises)
preexisting
prep, 3M
prepared and draped
prepatellar bursitis
press-fit design; stem
pressure
  compartmental
  manual
  tourniquet
pressure sore
pretendinous cord
pretibial edema
prickling
principle
  axial compression
  Enneking

Pritchard Mark II pin
Pritchard-Walker total elbow prosthesis
Pro-8 ankle brace
probe
  angled
  arthroscopic
  Bunnell
  dissecting
  intraosseous
  laser Doppler
  skin temperature monitoring
  ultrasonic
procedure (see *operation*)
procedure time
process
progression to full weightbearing
Prolene suture
proliferation, angiofibroblastic
prominence
  bony
  tibial tubercle
pronation and supination
prong, modified tonsil
prophylactic antibiotics
prophylactic anticoagulation
Proplast prosthesis
proprioception
prosthesis
  Aesculap-PM noncemented femoral
  AFI total hip replacement
  AHSC (Arizona Health Science
    Center-Volz) elbow
  Alivium implant metal
  AMC total wrist
  AML hip
  AML Tang femoral
  Amstutz cemented hip (TR-28)
  Anametric total knee
  anatomic surface
  APRL hand
  Arafiles elbow
  Arizona Health Science Center-Volz
    (AHSC) elbow
  Arthropor cup
  Attenborough knee
  Aufranc-Cobra hip

prosthosis *(cont.)*
 Aufranc-Turner cemented hip
 Austin Moore hip
 Autophor ceramic total hip
 Averett hip
 Bateman UPF II bipolar
 Bechtol hip
 Becker hand
 bicentric
 bicompartmental knee implant
 bicondylar knee
 Biofit press-fit acetabular
 Biomet
 Biometric
 Biophase implant metal
 Biotex implant metal
 bipolar femoral head
 bipolar hip replacement
 Blazina
 Bock knee
 Bombelli-Mathys-Morscher hip
 Brigham
 Bryan total knee implant
 Buchholz
 CAD femoral stem
 Calandruccio cemented hip
 Callender technique hip
 Calnan-Nicole
 capitellocondylar unconstrained
  elbow
 carpal lunate implant
 carpal scaphoid implant
 Cathcart Orthocentric hip
 Charnley cemented
 Charnley low friction hip
 Charnley-Müller hip
 Chatzidakis hinged Vitallium
  implant
 Chopart partial foot
 Christiansen hip
 Cintor knee
 Co-Cr-Mo (cobalt-chromium-
  tungsten-nickel) alloy
 Co-Cr-W-Ni (cobalt-chromium-
  tungsten-nickel) alloy
 Coballoy implant metal

prosthesis *(cont.)*
 Cofield shoulder
 cold-mold
 cold-weld
 collar-calcar support femoral
 Compartmental II
 compression-molded
 Conaxial ankle
 constrained hinged
 Contour internal
 Coonrad hinge
 Coonrad semiconstrained elbow
 custom-threaded
 DANA shoulder
 d'Aubigne femoral
 Dee totally constrained elbow
 De La Caffiniere trapeziometacarpal
 DePalma
 DePuy AML Porocoat stem
 DF80 (Wilson-Burstein) hip
 Dorrance hand
 Dow Corning Wright finger joint
 Dow Corning implant
 dual-lock hip
 Dupaco knee
 Dynaplex knee
 Eaton finger joint replacement
 Eicher femoral
 ELP femoral
 Englehardt femoral
 Ewald unconstrained elbow
 Exeter cemented hip
 femoral
 Fett
 finger joint implant
 Flatt finger joint
 Flatt finger/thumb
 forearm lift-assist
 four-bar linkage on knee
 Freeman-Samuelson
 Freeman-Swanson knee
 F.R. Thompson femoral
 fully constrained tricompartmental
  knee
 Galante hip
 Geomedic total knee

prosthesis *(cont.)*
  Geometric total knee
  Gerard
  Giliberty hip
  Gore-Tex knee
  great toe implant
  Gritti-Stokes knee
  GSB (Gschwind-Scheier-Bahler) elbow
  Gschwind-Scheier-Bahler (GSB) elbow
  Guepar hinged knee
  Gustilio hip
  HA 65101 implant metal
  Hamas
  Harris (HD-2) cemented hip
  Harris-CDH hip
  Harris-Galante hip
  Hastings hip
  Haynes-Stellite (HS) implant metal
  Hedley-Hungerford hip
  Henschke-Mauch SNS knee
  Herbert knee
  Hexcel knee
  HPS II hip
  Hunter tendon
  Hydra-Cadence knee
  ICLH ankle; knee
  Indiana conservative
  Indong Oh
  Insall-Burstein semiconstrained tricompartmental knee
  Iowa
  Ishizuki unconstrained elbow
  Jaffe-Capello-Averill hip
  Joplin toe
  Judet press-fit hip
  Kessler
  Kinematic fully constrained tricompartmental knee
  Kinematic II rotating hinge total
  Kirschner Medical Dimension knee
  Kudo unconstrained elbow
  Küntscher humeral

prosthesis *(cont.)*
  Lacey fully constrained tricompartmental knee
  LCS New Jersey knee prosthesis
  Leinbach femoral
  Lewis Trapezio
  Ling cemented hip
  Lippman hip
  Lisfranc below-knee
  Liverpool elbow
  London unconstrained elbow
  Lord press-fit hip
  low-neck femoral
  low-profile femoral
  Lowe-Miller unconstrained elbow
  Lunceford-Pilliar-Engh hip
  MacIntosh
  MacNab-English shoulder
  Mediloy implant metal
  madreporic hip
  manual locking knee
  Marmor modular knee
  Matchett-Brown cemented hip
  Mayo semiconstrained elbow
  Mazas totally constrained elbow
  McBride femoral
  McGehee elbow
  McKee-Farrar total hip
  McKeever Vitallium knee
  medium profile femoral metal
  Michael Reese articulated
  Miller-Galante hip
  Minneapolis
  Mittelmeier ceramic hip
  Mittlemeier noncemented femoral
  modular unicompartmental knee
  Monk hip
  Moore femoral; hip
  MP35N implant metal
  MST-6A1-4V
  Mueli wrist
  Müller dual-lock
  Müller total hip replacement
  NEB (New England Baptist) hip
  Neer shoulder (I and II)

prosthesis *(cont.)*
 Neer umbrella
 Neer Vitallium humeral
 New Jersey LCS knee
 Newton ankle
 Niebauer
 Noiles fully constrained tricompartmental knee
 nonhinged linked
 Normalize press-fit hip
 nudge control on
 Oh cemented hip
 Oh press-fit hip
 Optifix femoral
 Oregon Poly II ankle
 Orthochrome implant metal
 Ortholoc implant metal
 orthopedic
 Osteonics hip
 Overdyke hip
 patellar
 PCA unconstrained tricompartmental
 PCA unicompartmental knee
 Phoenix hip
 PMI-6A1-4V implant metal
 polycentric knee
 Poly-Dial
 polyethylene patellar implant
 Porocoated AML noncemented
 Porometal noncemented femoral
 porous coated hip
 press-fit condylar total knee
 press-fit implant
 Pritchard-Walker semiconstrained elbow
 Protasul-10 noncemented femoral
 Protasul-64 WF Zweymuller femoral
 provisional
 PTB supracondylar (SC)
 PTB suprapatellar (SP)
 PTS soft wedge
 radial head implant
 Richards Spectron metal-backed acetabular
 Ring total hip

prosthesis *(cont.)*
 Ringe hip
 RM isoelastic hip
 Robert Brigham total knee
 rotating hinge
 SACH (solid-ankle, cushioned heel) foot
 SAF (self-articulating femoral) hip replacement
 Sarmiento (STH-2) hip
 Sauerbach
 Sbarbaro hip
 Sbarbaro tibial plateau
 Schlein elbow
 Schlein semiconstrained elbow
 self-bearing ceramic hip
 semiconstrained tricompartmental knee
 Sharrard-Trentani
 Sheehan knee
 Sherfee
 Shier total knee
 Silastic radial head
 sintered implant
 Sinterlock implant metal
 Sivash hip
 SMA
 Smith ankle
 Smith-Petersen
 Souter unconstrained elbow
 Spectron hip
 Speed
 spherocentric fully constrained tricompartmental knee
 spherocentric knee
 S-ROM
 St. George-Buchholz ankle
 stainless steel implant metal
 Stanmore totally constrained elbow
 STD hip
 stemmed
 Stevens-Street elbow
 STH-2 (Sarmiento) hip
 Street-Stevens humeral
 Surgitek
 Swanson T-shaped great toe silastic

prosthesis *(cont.)*
    Syme amputation
    Syme foot
    Synatomic knee
    synthetic
    TARA (total articular replacement arthroplasty)
    TARA hip
    Tavernetti-Tennant
    Tharies hip replacement
    thermomechanical implant metal
    Thompson hip
    threaded titanium acetabular (TTAP)
    Thurst plate femoral
    tibial plateau
    Ti-Con
    Tillman
    Titan cemented hip
    titanium implant
    Tivanium implant metal
    Total Condylar Knee
    Total Condylar semiconstrained tricompartmental
    total hip replacement
    total joint replacement
    total knee replacement
    Townley TARA
    TPR ankle prosthesis
    trapezium implant
    Trapezoidal-28 hip
    trial
    Tri-Axial
    triaxial semiconstrained elbow
    Tri-Con
    tricompartmental knee
    Tri-Lock
    two-prong stem finger
    UCI ankle
    ulnar head implant
    unconstrained tricompartmental knee
    unicompartmental knee
    Universal hip
    UPF (universal proximal femur)
    Vanghetti

prosthesis *(cont.)*
    Varikopf
    Vinertia implant metal
    Vitallium-W implant metal
    Volz wrist
    Wadsworth unconstrained elbow
    Wagner
    Walldius knee
    Waugh knee
    Waugh total ankle replacement
    well-seated
    Whiteside knee
    Whiteside Ortholoc II condylar femoral
    William Harris hip
    Wilson-Burstein (DF80) hip
    wrist joint implant
    Xenophor femoral
    Young hinged knee
    Young-Vitallium hinged
    Zimalite implant metal
    Zimaloy implant metal
    Zimmer shoulder
prosthetic hook (see *hook*)
prosthetic support (see *support*)
prosthetist
Protasul implant metal
protector
    grooved
    Ortho-Foam
    PRN
protector splint
protein
    Bence Jones
    C-reactive
Protoplast cement
Protouch synthetic orthopedic padding
protractor
protrusio acetabuli
protrusion of the navicular
protrusion, disk
proximal carpal row
proximal focal femoral deficiency (PFFD)
proximally

PVNS = pigmented villonodular synovitis

pseudarthrosis
 congenital
 interspinous
pseudoarthrosis (see *pseudarthrosis*)
pseudoclaudication
pseudohypoparathyroidism
pseudoneuroma
psychomotor
PT (physical therapy)
PT (prothrombin time)
PTB (patellar tendon bearing) ankle-foot orthosis
PTB supracondylar (SC) prosthesis
PTB suprapatellar (SP) prosthesis
PTB-SC-SP prosthesis
PTS soft wedge prosthesis
PTT (partial thromboplastin time)
PTT (patellar tendon transfer)
pubic rami
pubic symphysis
puboischial area
Puddu tendon technique
Pugh sliding nail; plate; traction
pulley, cruciate
pulp, finger
pulsation
pulsing current (electrostimulation) for nonunion of fracture
Pulvertaft fishmouth stitch
pulvinar
pump bumps
pumps
 ankle
 knee
punch
 Acufex rotary
 bone
 cervical laminectomy
 Kerrison
 Schlesinger
 tibial
 tubular
purines, diet low in
purulent material
pus, puric
push-off by great toe

Putti arthrodesis; bone plast
Putti-Platt shoulder procedure
pyarthrosis
pylon attachment plate
pylon, metal
pyogenic granuloma
pyramidal tract

# Q, q

Q angle
quad (quadriceps)
quadrangle cartilage
quadratus femoris muscle; fascia
quadriceps apron
quadriceps wasting
quadricepsplasty
 Thompson
 V-Y
quadrilateral brim
quadriparesis
quadriplegia
quadropod cane
Queckenstedt sign
Quengel cast; hinge
Quenu nail plate removal technique
Quervain fracture
quiescence, quiescent

# R, r

rachialgia
rachicentesis
rachiocampsis
rachiochysis
rachiodynia

rachiokyphosis
rachiomyelitis
rachioparalysis
rachiopathy
rachioplegia
rachioscoliosis
rachiotomy
rachisagra
rachischisis
rachitic rosary sign
rachitomy
radial drift
radialized
radicular pain
radiculectomy
radiculitis
radiculoneuritis
radiculopathy
radioactive xenon clearance
radiocarpal
radiograph, plain film
radioisotope clearance assay
radiolucency, radiolucent
radiograph, radiography
radioscaphoid ligament
radioulnar subluxation
Radley-Liebig-Brown resection
RA (rheumatoid arthritis) factor
Raimiste sign
Rainbow cast sandal
raising
   crossed straight leg
   straight leg (SLR)
rales and rhonchi
Ralston-Thompson pseudarthrosis
   technique
ramus, rami
Ranawat-DeFiore-Straub technique
Rancho-type anklet foot control device
Raney-Crutchfield tong traction
range of excursion
range of motion (ROM)
   active (AROM)
   active and passive
   active-assisted
   passive

range of motion *(cont.)*
   restricted
rarefaction
rasp, raspatory
   Acufex convex
   Alexander
   angled
   Austin Moore
   Bacon
   carbon-tungsten
   Charnley
   Coryllos
   Cottle
   DePuy
   Fisher
   Putti bone
rasped, rasping
rate, sed (sedimentation)
Ratliff classification of avascular
   necrosis
Rauchfuss sling
ray
   long axis
   pollicized
Ray-Tec sponge
Raymond shoulder immobilizer
realign, realignment
ream, reamed, reaming
reamer
   acetabular
   Anspach
   Aufranc
   Austin Moore
   ball
   blunt tapered T-handled
   bone
   brace-type
   calcar
   Campbell
   cannulated Henderson
   chamfer
   Charnley
   Christmas tree
   conical
   corrugated
   cup

| reamer | 109 | reflex |

reamer *(cont.)*
  deepening
  DePuy
  expanding
  female
  fenestrated
  flexible medullary
  grater
  handle type
  Harris center-cutting acetabular
  hollow mill
  Indiana
  Küntscher
  male
  medullary canal
  Mira
  multisized
  Norton ball
  power
  rigid
  Rush awl
  Smith-Petersen
  spiral cortical
  spiral trochanteric
  step-cut
  T-handled
  tapered hand
  trochanteric
  Wagner acetabular
reanastomosis of blood supply to
  bone graft
reapproximation
recipient team
reconstruction (see also *operation*)
  five-one
  tenoplastic
recrudescence
rectus position
recurrent dislocation
Redi head halter
Redi-Around finger splint
Redi-Trac traction device
Redi-Vac cast cutter
Redigrip pressure bandage
reduce, reduction

reduction (see also *operation*)
  closed
  concentric
  open
  stable
  surgical
  trial
reduction of fracture
Reebok shoes
reefing procedure [handwritten: Reece shoe]
Reese dermatome
reevaluate, reevaluated
reexploration
refill, capillary
reflect, reflected
reflex, reflexes (see also *sign, test*)
  absent
  Achilles tendon
  adductor
  ankle
  Babinski
  Bekhterev-Mendel
  biceps
  Brain
  deep tendon
  delayed
  depressed
  dorsal
  elbow
  Hirschberg
  hyperactive
  knee jerk
  Mendel-Bekhterev
  motor
  muscle stretch
  patellar
  patelloadductor
  pathologic
  pectoral
  quadriceps
  radial
  Remak
  scapular
  scapulohumeral
  Stookey

reflex *(cont.)*
   stretch
   suprapatellar
   tendon
   toe
   triceps
   triceps surae
   ulnar
   von Bekhterev
refractory
Refsum syndrome
Regen flexion exercises
regeneration of nerve
rehabilitation
Reichenheim-King procedure
re-irrigation
Reiter syndrome
release of Dupuytren contracture
release (see also *operation)*
   adductor tendon and lateral
      capsular
   brevis
   capsular
   carpal tunnel
   fascial
   flexor-pronator origin
   key
   lateral capsular
   lateral retinaculum
   plantar plate
   retinacular
   soft tissue
   tendon
   trigger finger
   ulnar nerve
remodeling, bone
Renografin contrast media
repair (see also *operation)*
   ACL (anterior cruciate ligament)
   bone graft
   Bankart shoulder
   Boyd-Anderson biceps tendon
   Bunnell tendon
   DuVries hammertoe
   first-toe Jones
   five-one knee ligament

repair *(cont.)*
   fracture
   Kleinert
   MacNab shoulder
   primary
   rotator cuff
   Sever-L'Episcopo
   Staples-Black-Brostrom ligament
   Strickland tendon
   triad knee
   volar plate
   Watson-Jones (ankle fracture)
replacement (see *prosthesis)*
reprep and drape
Repro head halter
reroute
resection (see *operation)*
resection of meniscus
resector
   orthotome
   synovial
resin, polyacetal
resistance, strength against
resorption
   bone
   osteoclastic
rest, kidney
restorator
restrictor
   cement
   plastic marrow canal
retain, retained
reticulocytosis, cerebroside
retinaculum
   extensor
   patellar
retractor
   Adson cerebellum
   amputation
   appendiceal
   Beckman
   Bennett
   Blount anvil
   Blount knee
   Campbell
   Charnley pin

retractor *(cont.)*
    Charnley self-retaining
    cobra head-shaped
    curved
    Cushing
    double-ended right-angle
    double-hook Lovejoy
    Downey hemilaminectomy
    East-West
    Fahey
    Gelpi
    Hayes
    heavy-duty two-tooth
    Hibbs-type
    Hoen
    Hohmann
    Holscher knee; root
    humeral head
    Inge
    Israel
    Love root
    lower-hand
    Markham-Meyerding
    Mayo-Collins
    Meyerding
    mini-Hohmann
    Myers knee
    narrow-neck mini-Hohmann
    narrow-blade
    Ollier rake
    pin
    rake
    Richardson
    Rosenberg
    Sauerbruch
    Senn double-end
    sharp
    Sims
    skid humeral-head
    Smillie
    Sofield
    stiff ribbon
    Taylor
    two-prong rake
    U-shaped
    U.S.

retractor *(cont.)*
    upper-hand
    Volkman rake
    Wagner
    Weit-Arner
    Weitlander
    Wilson gonad
    Wink
re-treating
retrocalcaneal bursa
retroversion, femoral
revascularization of graft
revascularized tissue
Reverdin epidermal free graft
revision of total hip
revision, stump
Rezaian external fixation
rhabdomyoma
rhabdomyosarcoma, alveolar
rhachotomy
    Capener
    decompression
rheumatism, palindromic
rheumatoid arthritis (RA) factor
rheumatologist
Rhinelander pin
rhizomelic
rhizotomy (radicotomy)
rhonchus, rhonchi
rhythm, regular sinus
rib
    bicipital
    cervical
    false
    floating
    rudimentary
    slipping
    sternal
    true
    vertebral
rib belt orthosis
rib belt, Zim-Zap
Ribble bandage
rib contusion
rice bodies
Richards compression screw

Richardson retractor; rod
Richards Spectron metal-backed acetabular prosthesis
Riche-Cannieu anastomosis
Richet bandage
rickets
ridge
  greater multangular
  vastus lateralis
Ridlon plaster knife
right-hand dominant
rim, glenoid
Ring total hip prosthesis
ring
  doughnut
  drop-lock
  Fischer
  halo
  Ilizarov
  ischial weightbearing
  K-F (Kayser-Fleischer)
  orthosis drop-lock
  pelvic
  perichondral
  proximal-to-distal
Riordan tendon transfer technique
Riseborough-Radin classification of intercondylar fracture
Risser localizer scoliosis cast
Ritchie nail starter
RLE (right lower extremity)
RM isoelastic hip prosthesis
R/O (rule out)
Robert Brigham total knee prosthesis
Robert Jones dressing
Roberts technique
Robinnson-Chung-Farahvar clavicular morcellation
Robinson cervical spine fusion
Robinson-Riley cervical arthrodesis
Robinson-Southwick fusion technique
Rochester compression system
Rockwood classification of acromioclavicular injury
Rockwood-Green technique

rod
  compression
  Dacron-impregnated silicone
  distraction
  Ender
  fluted medullary
  Harrington
  Harris condylocephalic
  hinge
  Hunter silastic
  IM (intramedullary)
  Knodt
  Küntscher condylocephalic
  Luque
  Moe
  Mouradian
  Richardson
  Rush
  Sage
  Schneider
  Serrato forearm
  Stenzel
  straight threaded
  telescoping medullary
  telescopic
  threaded
  V-A alignment
  Wissinger
  Zickel
roentgenogram, two-plane
Roger Anderson compression device
Rogers cervical fusion technique
Rohadur
Rolando fracture
Rolator walker
rolfing (massage)
roll
  chest
  cotton
  hip
  radiolucent
  towel
Rolyan tibial fracture brace
ROM (range of motion)
Romberg sign; test

rongeur
  Adson
  angled jaw
  angled pituitary
  angular bone
  basket
  bayonet
  Beyer
  bone-nibbling
  Bruening-Citelli
  Campbell
  Colclough laminectomy
  curved bone
  disk
  double-action
  downbiting
  duckbill
  Ferris-Smith
  Kerrison down-biting
  Leksell
  pituitary
  Schlesinger cervical
  single action
  Spurling
  Stille
  Stille-Luer bone
  straight bone
  straight pituitary
  upbiting
  Leksell
room
  Allender vertical laminar flow
  Charnley laminar flow
Roos approach
root, nerve
Root-Siegal osteotomy
Rosenberg retractor
rotation
  external
  internal
  inward
  neutral
  outward
rotation-plasty, Van Ness
rotator
  external

rotator *(cont.)*
  internal
  long external
  short external
rotator cuff tear
rotoscoliosis
roughen the surface
roughening
rouleaux formation
Rousek extraction set
Roussy-Levy syndrome
Roux-duToit staple capsulorrhaphy
Roux-Goldthwait procedure
row, proximal carpal
Rowe disimpaction forceps
Rowe-Zarins shoulder immobilization technique
Rowland-Hughes splint
Royalite body jacket
Royle-Thompson transfer technique
rubber-shod (protected) clamp
Rubinstein-Taybi syndrome
rubor
RUE (right upper extremity)
Ruiz-Mora procedure
ruler, Berndt hip
Rumel aluminum splint
runner's bump
Rush driver-bender-extractor; nail
Russe bone graft
Russell traction for femoral fracture
Russell-Taylor interlocking nail
Russian forceps
Rust sign
Ryerson triple arthrodesis

# S, s

Sabel cast walker
sac
  bursal
  common dural
S-ROM prosthesis
SAC (short arm cast)
SACH (solid-ankle, cushioned heel) foot prosthesis
Sach nerve separator
sacralgia
sacralization
sacralized transverse process
Sacro-Eze lumbar support
sacroiliac (SI) joint
sacroiliac subluxation
sacroiliitis
sacrotuberous ligament
sacrovertebral angle
sacrum (sacral spine)
SAF (self-articulating femoral) hip replacement
Sage radial nail; rod
Sage-Clark technique
Sage-Salvatore classification of acromioclavicular joint injury
sagittal roll spondylolisthesis
Saha procedure
Saha transfer technique
Saint George (see *St. George*)
Sakellarides classification of calcaneal fracture
Salter fracture (I-VI); osteotomy
Salter-Harris classification
Saltiel brace
salts, gold
Salzer prosthesis
Samilson osteotomy
Sampson medullary nail
sandal, Rainbow cast
sandbag
Sanfilippo syndrome
sanguineous
Santa Casa distractor

Sarbo sign
sarcoid, Boeck
sarcoma
  alveolar soft part
  botryoid
  clear cell
  epithelioid
  Ewing
  high-grade surface osteogenic
  intracortical osteogenic
  low-grade central osteogenic
  malignant myeloid
  multicentric osteogenic
  osteogenic
  Paget associated osteogenic
  parosteal osteogenic
  postirradiation osteogenic
  reticulum cell
  small cell osteogenic
  synovial
Sarmiento (STH-2) hip prosthesis
Sarmiento short leg patellar tendon-bearing cast
sartorius tendon
Satterlee bone saw
saucerization
Sauerbach prosthesis
Savastano hemiknee
saw
  Adams
  Aesculap
  amputation
  bayonet
  Beaver
  Bishop
  Charriere bone
  circular
  Cottle
  counter rotating
  crosscut
  electric cast
  end-cutting reciprocating
  Engel plaster
  Gigli
  Hall air-driven oscillating
  Herbert

saw *(cont.)*
    Luck-Bishop bone
    oscillating
    power oscillating
    power-driven
    reciprocating motor
    sagittal surgical
    Satterlee bone
    single-blade
    twin-blade oscillating
    Zimmer oscillating
sawcut
saw guide (see *guide*)
Sayre splint; traction
Sbarbaro tibial plateau prosthesis
SBO (spina bifida occulta)
Scaglietti closed reduction technique
Scaglietti procedure scale, Harris hip
scalenus anticus muscle
scalloping of vertebrae
scalpel, Bard-Parker
scan
    bone
    CT (computerized tomographic)
    gallium
    radioisotope gallium
    radioisotope indium-labeled white blood cell
    radioisotope technetium
    technetium 99m diphosphonate
    technetium 99m pyrophosphate
    TSPP (technetium stannous pyrophosphate) rectilinear
    technetium 99m sulfur colloid
scanogram
scanography
scaphoid cookie in shoe
scaphoiditis
scapholunate
scapula, scapulae
    high-riding
    winged
scapular
scapulectomy
    Das Gupta
    Phelps

scapuloclavicular
scapulothoracic motion
scapulovertebral border
scar, scarred
Schaberg-Harper-Allen technique
Schanz angulation osteotomy
Schanz brace; collar; pin
Schauwecker patellar wiring technique
Scheie syndrome
Scheuermann disease
Schirmer test
Schlein elbow arthroplasty
Schlesinger cervical rongeur
Schmeisser spica
Schmidt rod holder
Schmorl node
Schneider driver-extractor; nail; rod
Schnute wedge resection technique
Schober test of lumbar flexion
Schreiber maneuver
Schrock procedure
Schutte basket, shovel-nose
Schwann tumor
schwannoma
Schweitzer spring plate
sciatic nerve irritation
sciatica
scintigraphy, bone
scissors
    Acufex
    arthroscopic
    blunt-tipped iris
    cartilage
    crown and collar
    curved Mayo
    Dean
    dissecting
    Mayo
    Metzenbaum
    Slip-N-Slip
    Smillie meniscus
    suture
scleroderma
sclerosing nonsuppurative osteitis
sclerosis, Monckeberg
sclerotic

scoliorachitis
scoliosis
  Cobb measurement of
  dextrorotary
  dextroscoliosis
  functional
  idiopathic
  levorotary
  levoscoliosis
  uncompensated rotary
  scoliosis correction with Dwyer cable
scope
  Doppler
  Harris
Scotchcast 2 casting tape
Scott glenoplasty technique
Scottish Rite hip orthosis
scout film
Scoville curet
screen, Lanex
screw
  AMBI hip
  AO cancellous
  AO cortex
  AO lag
  arthrodesis
  ASIF cancellous
  ASIF cortical
  Asnis cannulated
  Aten olecranon
  Basile
  Bechtol
  bicortical
  Bosworth
  buttress
  Calandruccio compression
  Campbell cannulated
  cancellous bone
  Carrell-Girard
  Collison
  compression hip
  compression lag
  cortical cancellous
  Coventry
  cruciate head
  cruciform

screw *(cont.)*
  DDT
  DeMuth
  double-threaded Herbert
  Duo-Driv
  Dwyer
  Eggers
  Geckler
  Glasgow
  Glass-Bessen transfixion
  Hamilton
  Henderson lag
  hex (hexagonal)
  hexagonal slot-cap
  hollow mill Asnis cannulated
  Howmedica ICS
  Johansson lag
  Jones
  Kaessmann
  Kristiansen eyelet lag
  lag
  Leinbach
  Lorenzo
  Lundholm
  malleolar
  Marion
  Martin
  McLaughlin
  mini AO
  Morris biphase
  Morris biplane
  Mouradian
  Neufeld
  NoLok
  Phillips
  Phillips head
  Phillips recessed head
  Richards
  Richards compression
  Rockwood
  Schanz
  self-tapping bone
  Shelton bone
  Sherman
  Simmons
  sliding compression hip

screw *(cont.)*
   stainless steel
   Steffe
   Stryker
   Swiss cancellous
   Synthes
   Thornton
   threaded cancellous
   thumb
   titanium
   Townley
   Townsend-Gilfillan
   transfixion
   varus-valgus adjustment
   Venable-Stuck
   Vitallium
   Wagner-Schanz
   wood
   Woodruff
   Zimmer compression hip
   Zuelzer
screwdriver
   automatic
   Becker
   Cardan
   collet adapter
   Collison
   cross-slot
   cruciform
   Flatt self-retaining
   Ken
   Phillips head
   self-retaining
   single-slot
   torque
   Williams
screw fixation
screw head
   countersink
   Phillips
screw-in ceramic acetabular cup
screw-plate
   Calandruccio impaction
   Zimmer impaction
scrub
   Betadine

scrub *(cont.)*
   Hibiclens
Scuderi technique
scultetus bandage
seat, ischial-bearing
seated, properly
sed (sedimentation) rate
Seddon technique
sedentary lifestyle
segmental bone loss
Segond fracture
Seinsheimer classification of femoral fracture
self-inflicted gunshot wound
self-retaining screwdriver
Sell-Frank-Johnson extensor shift technique
semilunar bone
semitendinosus tendon
Senn double-end retractor
sensation
   altered
   catching
   diminished
   light touch
   phantom
   pinprick
   return of
   touch
   vibration
sense, joint position
sensorimotor
sensory or motor deficit
separation, AC (acromioclavicular)
separator, Sach nerve
sepsis, septic
septum, intermuscular
sequela, sequelae
sequester, sequestered, sequestration
sequestrectomy
sequestrum
SER-IV (supination, external rotation—type IV) fracture
Series-II humeral head
serosanguineous
serration

Serrato forearm pin; rod
sesamoid
  accessory
  bipartite
sesamoidectomy
sessile
set
  acetabular trial
  AO minifragment
  Hollywood bed extension hook
  nail
  Rousek extraction
set angle of toes
Seton hip brace
setter, bone plug
Sever disease
Sever modification of Fairbank
  technique
Sever-L'Episcopo repair of shoulder
SEWHO (shoulder-elbow-wrist-hand
  orthosis)
shaft
  distal third
  middle third
  ministem
  proximal third
shank, steel
Shanz dressing
Sharpey fibers
Sharrard transfer technique
Sharrard-Trentani prosthesis
shaver
  automated
  Dyonics
  motorized meniscus
  motorized suction
  synovial
shaving
  arthroscopic
  femoral condylar
shears
  Brunn plaster
  Esmarch plaster
  Hercules plaster
  Stille plaster

sheath
  arthroscope
  muscle
  synovial
  tendon
Sheehan knee prosthesis
sheet
  laparotomy
  sterile
Sheffield hand elevator; support
shelf
  Blumer
  lateral
  medial
  patellar
shelling off of cartilage
Shelton femur fracture classification
shelving
Shenton line
Shepherd fracture
Sherfee prosthesis
Sherk-Probst technique
Sherman bone plate; block test
shield, arthroscopic
Shiers total knee prosthesis
Shifrin wire twister
shift
  pivot
  plantar
shod, rubber
shoe, shoes
  Bebax (for forefoot deformity)
  Bevin
  cut-out
  extended-counter
  high heel
  infant clown cast
  Moon Boot
  narrow toebox
  normal last
  open-toe
  orthopedic oxford
  pointed toe
  PRN
  Reebok
  Plastizote

shoe *(cont.)*
  reverse last
  rocker
  soft-vamp
  space
  straight last
  tarsal pronator
  torque heel
  Vibram rockerbottom
  Viva
  WACH orthopedic
  wedge adjustable cushioned heel
    (WACH)
  wide toebox
  wooden-soled
shoe cookie
shoe extension, Legg-Perthes
shoe filler
shoe insert
  cushioned
  UCB
shoe lift
shoe wear, abnormal
short head of biceps
shortening
  Achilles tendon
  leg
shoulder immobilizer (see *immobilizer*)
shoulder, Little Leaguer's
shoulder pointer
shoulder prosthesis (see *prosthesis*)
shoulder repair (see *repair*)
shoulder spica cast
shoulder, apprehension
Shriner pin
shrinker, stump
Shriver-Johnson interphalangeal
  arthrodesis
shucking
SI (sacroiliac) joint
sickle cell anemia
sideswipe elbow fracture
sidewall
Siffert-Forster-Nachamie arthrodesis
Siffert-Storen intraepiphyseal
  osteotomy

sign
  Adson
  Allen
  Allis
  Amoss
  Anghelescu
  antecedent
  anterior drawer
  anterior tibial
  anvil
  Apley
  apprehension
  Babinski
  Barlow
  bayonet
  Beevor
  bowstring
  Bragard
  Brudzinski
  Bryant
  Burton
  camelback
  Cantelli
  Chaddock
  choppy sea
  Chvostek
  Cleeman
  Codman
  cogwheel
  commemorative
  Comolli
  contralateral
  Coopernail
  crescent
  Dawbarn
  Dejerine
  Demianoff
  Desault
  double camelback
  drawer
  Dupuytren
  Egawa
  Erichsen
  fabere (flexion, abduction, external
    rotation, extension)

sign *(cont.)*
   fadir (flexion, adduction, internal rotation)
   Fajersztajn crossed sciatic
   fan
   Finkelstein
   Fleck
   Fränkel
   Friedreich
   Froment paper
   Gaenslen
   Gage
   Galant
   Galeazzi
   Goldthwait
   Gower
   Guilland
   Hawkins
   head-at-risk
   Helbing
   Hirschberg
   Hoffman
   Homans
   hot-cross-bun skull
   Hueter
   Huntington
   J
   Jenet
   Kanavel
   Keen
   Kellgren
   Kernig
   Kerr
   Langoria
   Lasègue
   Laugier
   Leichtenstern
   Leri
   Lhermitte
   Linder
   long tract
   Lorenz
   Ludloff
   Maisonneuve
   Marie-Foix
   McMurray

sign *(cont.)*
   Mendel-Bekhterev
   Mennell
   Minor
   Morquio
   Morton-Horwitz nerve cross-over
   movie
   Naffziger
   Nelson
   Oppenheim
   Ortolani
   pathognomonic
   Payr
   Piotrowski
   piston (on x-ray)
   pivot-shift
   pronation
   pseudo-Babinski
   Queckenstedt
   rachitic rosary
   radialis
   Raimiste
   Riordan
   Romberg
   Rust
   Sarbo
   Schlesinger
   Soto-Hall
   Speed
   spine
   stairs
   Strümpell
   Strunsky
   theater
   Thomas
   thorn
   Thurston-Holland
   tibialis
   Tinel
   toe
   toe spread
   Turyn
   Vanzetti
   Voshell
   Wartenberg
   windshield wiper (on x-ray)

sign *(cont.)*
  Yergason
Sigvaris stocking
Silastic radial head prosthesis; drain
Silesian bandage prosthetic support
Silfverskiöld lengthening technique
Silfverskiöld test
silicone gel
silk, Owens
Silver bunionectomy
Simmonds-Menelaus metatarsal
  osteotomy
Simmons Vari-Hite orthopedic bed
Simplex P bone cement
Simpson sugar-tong splint
Sims retractor
Sinding-Larsen-Johansson disease
Singh index of osteoporosis
sinogram
sintering
Sinterlock implant metal
sinus
  osteomyelitic
  pilonidal
site
  donor
  fracture
  nonunion of fracture
  operative
  recipient
Sivash hip prosthesis
sizer
Sjögren syndrome
skeletal defects
skeletally mature
skeleton, bony
skeletonize, skeletonized
skeletonizing
skewer, skewering
skid
  bone
  hip
  Murphy-Lane bone
Skil Saw
Skillern fracture
skin blood flow determination

skive (shave), skived
Skoog procedure for release of
  Dupuytren contracture
Slätis pelvic fracture frame
SLC (short leg cast)
SLE (systemic lupus erythematosus)
sleeve
  circumferential ligamentous
  drill
  obturator
sling
  Barton
  collar-and-cuff
  cradle arm
  envelope-type arm
  Glisson
  Haacker
  Kenny Howard shoulder
  Kodel knee
  Legg-Perthes
  Pavlik
  pelvic
  Rauchfuss
  rubber
  Slingers arm
  stockinette
  Teare
  triangular
  Velpeau
  Vogue arm
  Weil
sling-and-swath bandage
Slingers arm sling
slip of tendon
Slip-N-Snip scissors
sliver of bone
Slocum lateral pivot-shift test
slough, skin
SLR (straight leg raising)
SLRT (straight leg raising test)
SLWC (short leg walking cast)
SMA prosthesis
Smillie-Beaver blade
Smith-Davis Converta-Hite
  orthopedic bed
Smith-Petersen nail with Lloyd adapter

SMo (stainless steel and molybdenum)
snap, snapping
snapping hip
snuffbox, anatomical
snug, snugged, snugging
soap, Betadine
sock
    cast
    Spandex Lycra three-ply stump
    stump
socket
    check
    Poly-Dial
    quadrilateral
    total contact
Sofield osteotomy
soft tissue plication
Somerville procedure
SOMI (skull-occiput-mandibular immobilization) orthosis
SOMI (sterno-occipital-mandibular immobilizer) brace
Sorbie classification of calcaneal fracture
Sorbothane heel cushions
sore, pressure
Soto-Hall bone graft
sound, tearing
Souter unconstrained elbow prosthesis
Southwick biplane osteotomy
Southwick-Robinson anterior cervical approach
space
    dead
    disk
    epidural
    first web
    increased lateral joint
    intercondylar (ICS)
    lateral joint
    popliteal
    web
spacer
    acetabular
    joint
spacer-tensor jig IV

Spandex Lycra three-ply stump sock
Spanko shoe insert
spasm
    muscle
    paraspinal muscle
    paravertebral muscle
spastic gait
Spectron hip prosthesis
Speed V-Y muscle-plasty
Speed-Boyd radial-ulnar technique
Spherocentric fully constrained tricompartmental knee prosthesis
spica cast; splint (see *cast*)
Spiegleman acromioclavicular splint
Spier elbow arthrodesis
spike of bone
spike, Gissane
spina bifida occulta (SBO)
spinal column
spinal fusion (see *fusion; operation*)
spinal instability
spine
    cervical (C)
    Charcot
    coccygeal (coccyx)
    dorsal (D)
    iliac
    ischial
    kissing
    lumbar (L)
    lumbosacral (LS)
    mandibular
    maxillary
    nasal
    poker
    posterior-inferior
    sacral (S)
    thoracic (T)
    thoracolumbar
    trochanteric
spinoglenoid notch
spinothalamic tract
Spira procedure
Spittler procedure
spline
    Blount

spline *(cont.)*
  Bosworth
  flat
  Rowland-Hughes
splint (see also *bar; orthosis*)
  Abbott
  abduction
  abduction humeral
  acrylic template
  Adam and Eve
  Adams
  adjustable
  aeroplane (also airplane)
  Agnew
  air pressure
  airfoam
  airplane (also aeroplane)
  Alumafoam
  aluminum bridge
  aluminum fence
  aluminum foam
  anchor
  Anderson
  angle
  anterior
  any-angle
  Aquaplast
  Asch
  Ashhurst
  balanced
  Balkan
  ball-peen
  banjo
  Barlow cruciform infant
  baseball finger
  Basswood
  Bavarian
  Baylor
  Bloom
  Böhler
  Böhler-Braun
  Bond
  Bowlby
  bracketed
  Brady leg
  Brant aluminum

splint *(cont.)*
  Buck
  buddy
  Bunnell knuckle-bender
  Bunnell outrigger
  Burnham thumb and finger
  Cabot posterior
  Campbell
  cap
  Capner
  Carl P. Jones traction
  Carter
  Chandler felt collar
  Chatfield-Girdlestone
  clavicle
  clavicular cross
  Clayton greenstick
  clubfoot
  coaptation
  cock-up hand
  Colles
  Comforfoam
  countertraction
  Craig
  Cramer
  Cramer wire
  Culley
  Curry
  Davis
  Delbet
  Denis Browne clubfoot
  DePuy open spindle
  dorsal
  drop foot
  Dupuytren
  Duran-Houser wrist
  Dyna knee
  dynamic
  Eaton
  Eggers
  elephant-ear clavicle
  Englemann
  Erich
  extension block(ing)
  felt collar
  fence

splint *(cont.)*
  Ferciot tiptoe
  Fillauer night
  finger
  finger cot
  forearm
  Forrester
  Foster
  Fox
  Frac-Sur
  Frejka pillow
  frog
  Fruehevald
  Funsten
  Gagnon
  Gibson
  Gilmer
  Gooch
  Gordon
  Granberry
  Gunning
  gutter
  half-shell
  hallux valgus night
  Hammond
  Hanna night
  Harrington outrigger
  Hart
  Haynes-Griffin
  hinged cylinder
  Hirschtick
  Hodgen
  Ilfield-Gustafson
  inflatable
  Jelanko
  Joint Jack finger
  Jonell
  Jones
  Joseph
  Kanavel cock-up
  Karfoil
  Kazanjian
  Keller-Blake half ring
  Kerr
  Keystone
  knuckle bender-type

splint *(cont.)*
  Lambrinudi
  Levis
  Lewin baseball finger
  Lewin-Stern
  Liston
  live
  long arm
  long leg
  loop-lock cock-up
  Love
  Lytle
  Magnuson
  Mason-Allen universal
  Mayer
  McGee
  McIntire
  McLeod
  Middeldorpf
  Mohr
  molded posterior plaster
  Murray-Jones
  Murray-Thomas
  Neubeiser
  night
  O'Donaghue
  Oppenheimer spring wire
  orthoplastic
  outrigger
  padded tongue blade
  Pavlik
  Peabody
  pelvic
  Phelps
  pillow
  plaster
  polyvinylalcohol
  Pond adjustable
  Ponseti
  Postalume finger
  posterior
  Pott
  protecto
  Putti
  quick
  Redi-Around finger

splint *(cont.)*
   Roger Anderson
   Rowland-Hughes
   Rumel aluminum
   safety pin
   Sayre
   Scott
   shin
   short arm
   short leg
   shoulder spica
   Simpson sugar-tong
   Slocum
   Speed
   spica
   Spiegleman acromioclavicular
   Stader
   static
   Stax finger
   stirrup plaster
   Strampelli
   Stromeyer
   Stuart Gordon
   sugar-tong plaster
   Swanson hand
   Tauranga
   Taylor
   Thomas hinged
   Thomas suspension
   Thompson
   thumb web
   Tobruk
   Toronto
   traction
   triangular pillow
   universal gutter
   Valentine
   Velcro
   Vesely-Street
   volar plaster
   Volkmann
   von Rosen cruciform
   Weil
   well leg
   Wertheim
   Wilson

splint *(cont.)*
   wraparound
   yucca wood
   Zimfoam
   Zimmer
   Zucker
splint attachment, Pearson
splinted in position of function
splinter
splinting
   night
   pelvic
split Russell skeletal traction
spondylalagia
spondylarthritis
spondylarthrocace
spondylexarthrosis
spondylitis deformans
spondylitis, ankylosing
spondylizema
spondylodynia
spondylolisthesis
   sagittal roll
   slip angle
spondylolysis
spondylomalacia
spondylopathy
spondylopyosis
spondyloschisis
spondylosis
spondylosyndesis
spondylotomy
sponge
   gauze
   lap (laparotomy)
   Mikulicz
   Ray-Tec
   Vistec
spongy appearance
Sponsel oblique osteotomy
sprain
spread, Fowler
spreader
   Beeson cast
   Hoffer-Daimler cast
   lamina

Sprengel deformity
spring, Weiss
spring-loaded lock on orthosis
spur
    acromial
    bone
    heel
    traction
Spurling rongeur; test
spurring
    anterior
    inferior
squatting ability
S-ROM prosthesis
St. George-Buchholz ankle prosthesis
St. Vitus dance
stability
    lateral
    ligamentous
stabilize, stabilized, stabilization
stabilizer
stable to motion
stable, stability
Stack shoulder procedure
Stader pin; splint
Stagnara wake-up test
Staheli shelf procedure
stairs, trouble ascending and descending
stairstep-type fracture
Stamm procedure for intra-articular hip fusion
stamps, Gelfoam
Stanisavljevic technique
Stanmore shoulder arthroplasty
staple
    automatic
    barb
    Blount
    Coventry
    Day
    Downing
    duToit
    epiphyseal
    Howmedica Vitallium
    Johannesberg

staple *(cont.)*
    O'Brien
    osteoclast tension
    Owestry
    skin
    Stone four-point
    tabletop Stone
    Vitallium
    Zimaloy
staple gun
Staples elbow arthrodesis
Staples-Black-Broström ligament repair
stapling
    Blount
    epiphyseal
starch bandage
Stark-Moore-Ashworth-Boyes technique
starter, Ritchie nail
static fixation
static locking nail
station and gait
station test
status post
status
    ambulatory
    intact neurovascular
Stax finger splint
STD hip prosthesis
steel shank
Steel triple innominate osteotomy
Steffe plates and screws for lumbar fusion
Steindler flexorplasty
Steindler stripping technique
Steinmann pin with Crowe pilot point
stellate sympathetic ganglion block
stem
    Aufranc-Turner
    fenestrated
    Harris-Galante
    Moore
    nonfenestrated
    press-fit
    regular
    roundback
    straight

stem *(cont.)*
　trial
　Zimmer bone
stem base plate
stemmed prosthesis
stenosing tenosynovitis
stenosis, spinal
stent dressing
Stenzel rod
step cutting
step-cut transection
Steri-Strips
sterile 4 x 4's
sterile saline solution
steroids, tapering dose
sternoclavicular joint
sternocleidomastoid muscle
steroid myopathy
Stevens-Street elbow prosthesis
Stewart-Harley ankle arthrodesis
Stewart-Morel syndrome
STH-2 (Sarmiento) hip prosthesis
Stickler syndrome
Stieda fracture
stiff-man syndrome
stiffness, joint
Stiles-Bunnell transfer technique
Still disease
Stille-Liston bone-cutting forceps
Stille-Luer bone rongeur
stimulation
　electric
　electrical surface
　galvanic
　magnetic
　transcutaneous electrical nerve
　　(TENS)
stimulator
　battery-pack
　constant direct current
　dorsal column
　EBI bone
　Osteo-Stim bone
stippling
stirrups, traction
stitch (see *suture*)

stock, poor bone
stockinette
　basket
　bias
　bias-cut
　tubular
stockinette cut on the bias
stockinette, and sling and swath
stocking
　antiembolism
　Jobst
　long leg
　Orthawear antiembolism
　Sigvaris
　TED
Stone four-point staple
storiform pattern
Storz arthroscope
straight leg raising test
strain, muscle
Strampelli splint
strap
　capsular
　Chopart patellar
　crotch
　Meek clavicle
　suspension
　Velcro
strap muscles
Strayer tendon technique
Street-Stevens humeral prosthesis
strength
　extrinsic muscle
　fatigue
　5/5
　hand grasp
　hand grip
　intrinsic muscle
　motor
　tensile
　yield
strength against resistance
stress
　hyperextension
　mediolateral
　shear

stress *(cont.)*
  valgus
  varus
  Strickland tendon repair
  stripper
    Brand tendon
    Bunnell tendon
    cartilage
    tendon
  Stromeyer splint
  structures, lateral supporting
  Strümpell sign
  Strunsky sign
  strut graft
  strut-type pin
  Struthers
    arcade of
    ligament of
  Stryker fracture frame
  Stryker Surgilav machine
  STSG (split-thickness skin graft)
  Stuart Gordon splint
  stud, fixation
  study
    Doppler
    electromyographic
    kinematic
    nerve conduction
    tension-to-failure
stump shrinker, elastic
styloid, radial
styloidectomy, Stewart
stylus, marking
Styrofoam filler block
subacromial bursa
subcapital fracture
subchondral plate
subclavian steal syndrome
subcoracoid shoulder dislocation
subcutaneous fasciotomy
subcuticular closure
subfascial transposition
subglenoid shoulder dislocation
sublux, subluxed, subluxated
subluxation
subluxing patella
subperiosteal fracture
subperiosteally
subsartorial tunnel
subscapularis muscle
subtalar articulation
subtotal meniscectomy
subtrochanteric fracture
subungual abscess
suction tip
  Frazier
  neurosurgical
suction tube, Adson
suction-irrigation system
Sudeck atrophy; disease
sugar-tong splint
Sugioka transtrochanteric osteotomy
sulcus angle
Superglue (cyanoacrylate)
Superior Sleeprite Hi-Lo orthopedic
  bed
superolaterally
superomedial portal
supination
support
  Arizona leg
  bed cradle
  billet prosthetic
  condylar cuff prosthetic
  fork strap prosthetic
  Friedman elbow
  Fromison elbow
  Houston halo cervical
  Kerr-Lagen abdominal
  OEC wrist/forearm
  open patella knee
  Philadelphia collar cervical
  Sacro-Eze lumbar support
  Sheffield hand
  Silesian bandage prosthetic
  standard U patellar
  waist belt prosthetic
suppuration, suppurative
supraclavicular region
supracondylar varus osteotomy
supramalleolar osteotomy
suprapatellar plica

supraspinatus tendon
sural nerve
surcingle, Von Lackum
surface(s)
  acetabular weightbearing
  apposing articular
  articular
  bleeding bone
  bone
  bosselated
  cartilaginous joint
  contiguous articular
  endosteal
  joint
  roughened articular
  weightbearing
Surfit adhesive
Surgairtome
surgery (see *operation*)
surgibone, Boplant
Surgical Simplex P radiopaque bone cement
surgical site
Surgilav machine
Surgitek prosthesis
suspension
  adjustable Thomas splint
  balanced
  finger-trap
  half-ring Thomas splint
  overhead
  sling
  Thomas splint
suspension, balanced
sustentaculum tali
Sutherland-Greenfield double innominate osteotomy
Sutter-CPM knee device
suture (also called *stitch*)
  apical
  bundle
  Bunnell wire pull-out; crisscross
  buried
  catgut
  chromated
  chromic

suture *(cont.)*
  circular wire
  clove-hitch
  compression stay
  Dermalon
  Dexon
  Donati
  Ethibond
  Ethiflex
  Ethilon
  figure-of-8
  Gillies
  guy
  horizontal mattress
  interrupted
  intracuticular
  intradermal
  inverted
  Kessler
  mattress
  Maxon
  McLaughlin modification of Bunnell pull-out
  Mersilene
  modified Kessler
  monofilament nylon
  near-far
  nonabsorbable
  Nurolon
  nylon
  plain gut
  plastic
  Polydek
  Prolene
  pull-out wire
  Pulvertaft fishmouth
  running
  simple
  stainless steel
  subcutaneous
  subcuticular
  swaged-on
  tack
  Tevdek
  transfixion
  Tycron

*Swedo ankle brace*

| suture | 130 | syndrome |

suture *(cont.)*
  undyed
  vertical mattress
  Vicryl
  wire
swaged
swan-neck deformity
Swanson Convex condylar arthroplasty
Swanson Silastic prosthesis
Swanson T-shaped great toe silastic prosthesis
swath (noun); swathe (verb)
SWD (short wave diathermy)
Swedish knee cage orthosis; portal
swelling
  boggy
  joint
swing phase control
Swiss cancellous screw
Syme amputation, Wagner modification of
symphysis pubis
symptomatology
symptoms, functionally debilitating
synarthrosis
synathresis
Synatomic knee prosthesis
synchondrosis
synchondrotomy
syndactyly
syndesmectomy
syndesmopexy
syndesmoplasty
syndesmorrhaphy
syndesmosis, tibiofibular
syndesmotomy
syndrome
  adrenogenital
  Aicardi
  Albright
  Albright-McCune-Sternberg
  anterior cervical cord
  anterior compartment
  anterior tibial compartment
  Apert
  Arnold-Chiari

syndrome *(cont.)*
  Babinski-Fröhlich
  bicipital
  black heel
  blue toe
  broad thumb-big toe
  Brown-Séquard
  carpal tunnel
  cauda equina
  central cord
  clenched fist
  compartment
  cord traction
  Cornelia de Lange
  cubital tunnel
  de Lange
  Dejerine-Sottas
  diffuse idiopathic skeletal hyperostosis (DISH)
  Down
  Ehlers-Danlos
  entrapment
  Fanconi
  filum terminale
  flexor origin
  Goldenhar
  Guillain-Barré
  hammer digit
  Hunter
  impingement
  Jarcho-Levin
  Klinefelter
  Klippel-Feil
  Klippel-Trenaunay
  Larson
  Maffucci
  Marfan
  Maroteaux-Lamy
  milk-alkali
  Milkman
  Morel
  Morquio
  Naffziger
  nail-patella
  naviculocapitate fracture
  patellar malalignment

syndrome (cont.)
　Poland
　Refsum
　Reiter
　Roussy-Levy
　Rubinstein-Taybi
　Sanfilippo
　scalenus anticus
　Scheie
　Sinding-Larsen-Johansson
　Sjögren
　Stewart-Morel
　Stickler
　stiff-man
　subclavian steal
　superior mesenteric artery
　TAR (thrombocytopenia—absent radius)
　tarsal tunnel
　tensor fasciae latae
　thoracic outlet
　Tietze
　Turner
　ulnar nerve entrapment
　ulnar tunnel
synostosis
　cervical
　congenital radioulnar
synovectomy, Albright (hip)
synovia
synovial fringe
synovial frond
synovial plica
synoviochondromatosis
synoviogram
synovioma
synovitis
　boggy
　disseminated-type pigmented villonodular
　florid
　hypertrophic
　parapatellar
　pigmented villonodular
　proliferative
　rheumatoid arthritis

synovitis (cont.)
　villonodular
　villous
synovium, opaque
Synthes compression hip screw
Synthes plate; wire guide
synthetic prosthesis
syringomyelia
system
　Anametric knee
　Andersson hip status
　APR total hip system
　ASIF
　Bassett electrical stimulation
　Bowden cable suspension
　Brighton electrical stimulation
　cable suspension
　cannulated guided hip screw
　Charnley total hip
　cruciate condylar knee
　d'Aubigne hip status
　double inflow cannula
　Dwyer-Wickham electrical stimulation
　EBI bone healing
　Ewald elbow arthroplasty rating
　Fowler knee
　Freeman-Swanson knee
　Geomedic
　Harris hip status
　haversian
　Howmedica knee
　Inglis-Pellicci elbow arthroplasty rating
　Iowa hip status
　Judet hip status
　Larson hip status
　Mazur ankle rating
　Morrey elbow arthroplasty rating
　PCA primary total knee
　PCA universal total knee instrument
　Polycentric and Wide-Track knee
　Postel hip status
　posterior cruciate condylar knee
　Rochester compression

system *(cont.)*
    Russell-Taylor interlocking
      medullary nail
    Savastano Hemi-Knee
    Spherocentric knee
    suction-irrigation
    Total Condylar Knee
    Townley anatomic knee
    unicompartmental knee
    Unicondylar Geomedic Hemi-Knee
    variable axis knee
    Wisconsin compression
systemic lupus erythematosus (SLE)

# T, t

T bar guide
T buttress plate
T condylar fracture
T fashion
T fracture
T handle trocar
T-handled hook; reamer
T nail, Delitala
T plate
T-shaped AO plate
T-shaped inserter
T-spine (thoracic spine)
T splint
tabes dorsalis
tabetic foot
table
    Albee-Compere fracture
    Bell
    Burstein cast
    Chick fracture
    fluoroscopic
    fracture
    Green-Anderson growth
    inner
    Sieman

table *(cont.)*
    Stryker surgical hand
    tilting
table extension, Maquet
tabletop Stone staple
tablet, bonemeal
taboparesis
Tachdjian hamstring lengthening
tactile anesthesia
tailbone
tailor, tailored
takeoff
talar dome
talectomy
talipes calcaneovalgus
talipes calcaneus
talipes cavus
talipes equinovalgus
talipes equinovarus
talipes equinus
talipes, flexible
talocalcaneal coalition
talocalcaneonavicular articulation
talometatarsal angle
talus
    beaking of head of
    congenital vertical
    vertical
tamp, bone
tangential x-ray view
tank, Hubbard physical therapy
tap
    AO
    synovial
tape
    bias-cut
    graded Gore-Tex
    Mersilene
    TufStuf II cast
    umbilical
tapering dose steroids
TAR (thrombocytopenia—absent
    radius) syndrome
TARA (total articular resurfacing
    arthroplasty)

targeting bead
tarsal coalition
tarsometatarsal articulation
tarsonavicular
Tauranga splint
Tavernetti-Tennant knee prosthesis
Taylor back brace
Taylor-Daniel-Weiland technique
Taylor-Knight brace
TCL (tibial collateral ligament)
TCO (total contact orthosis)
TCPM pneumatic tourniquet system
tear
   anterior horn meniscal
   bucket-handle
   cleavage
   degenerative
   horizontal
   iatrogenic
   interstitial
   meniscal
   midsubstance
   parrot-beak
   posterior horn meniscal
   radial
   ratty meniscal
   rotator cuff
Teare sling
tearing sound
technetium 99m diphosphonate
technetium 99m pyrophosphate
technetium 99m scan
technetium 99m sulfur colloid scan
technetium bone scan
technetium labeled methylene diphosphonate
technique (see *operation*)
TED (thromboembolic disease) hose; stockings
Tegaderm dressing
Tegtmeier elevator
telangiectatic osteosarcoma
Telectronic electrical stimulation device
Telfa dressing; gauze
Temper-Foam

template
   acetabular cup
   femoral condylar
   malleable
   Moore
   prosthesis
templating
tibial track
transparent
Temple University nail; plate
tenderness
   joint line
   percussion
   point
   rebound
tendinitis
tendinous attachment
tendo Achillis mechanism
tendon
   abductor
   accessory communicating
   Achilles
   adductor
   aponeurotic
   brachial plexus
   brachioradialis
   calcaneal
   carpi radialis brevis
   common
   conjoined
   EHL (extensor hallucis longus)
   gracilis
   infraspinatus
   midpatellar
   obturator internus
   palmaris longus
   patellar
   patelloquadriceps
   popliteal
   quadriceps
   sartorius
   semitendinosus
   slip of
   snapping
   supraspinatus
tendon repair (see *repair*)

tendon transfer (see *operation*)
tendon tucker
  Bishop-Black
  Bishop-DeWitt
  Bishop-Peter
  Burch-Greenwood
tendosynovitis
tenectomy
tenodesis
  Eggers
  Fowler
  MacIntosh extra-articular
  Norwood
  Westin
tenodynia
tenolysis
tenomyoplasty
tenomyotomy
tenonectomy
tenontagra
tenontomyotomy
tenontophyma
tenontothecitis
tenophyte
tenoplasty
tenorrhaphy
tenosuspension
tenositis
tenostosis
tenosynovectomy
tenosynovitis, stenosing
tenotomized
tenotomy
  adductor
  Braun
  extensor
  Z-plasty
tenotomy of metatarsophalangeal joint
TENS (transcutaneous electrical nerve stimulation) unit
TENS-Pac
Tensilon test for myasthenia gravis
tension band wiring technique
tension forces
tension, tensioned
tensioner, Dwyer

tensor fasciae latae (TFL) syndrome
teres, ligamentum
test (see also *maneuver; sign*)
  abduction stress
  Achilles squeeze
  Addis
  adduction stress
  Allen
  ANA (antinuclear antibody)
  ankle jerk reflex
  anterior drawer
  anteroposterior stress
  antinuclear antibody (ANA)
  anvil
  Apley grinding
  apprehension
  axial compression
  axial load
  Barlow
  Bekhterev
  bench
  biceps jerk reflex
  bracelet
  British
  Callaway
  Chiene
  chin-to-chest
  Coleman block
  compression
  contralateral straight leg raising
  Cozen
  Doppler bidirectional
  dual-photon densitometry (for osteoporosis)
  duck waddle (of knee joints and menisci)
  Dugas
  Duncan prone rectus
  EAST (external rotation, abduction stress test)
  elbow jerk reflex
  Ely
  external rotation, abduction stress (EAST)
  external rotation recurvatum
  fabere (flexion, abduction, external rotation)

test (cont.)
  fadir (flexion, adduction, internal rotation)
  Fairbanks apprehension
  Favort and Feder
  femoral nerve stretch
  femoral nerve traction
  finger-to-nose
  Finkelstein
  flexion-rotation-drawer
  foot placement
  Fournier
  Gaenslen
  gluteus maximus tensing
  gracilis
  grimace
  grinding
  Hamilton ruler
  heel-to-shin
  heel-palm
  Hughston external rotation recurvatum
  Hughston knee jerk
  Hughston-Losee jerk
  hyperextension
  iliac compression
  Ingram-Withers-Speltz motor inhibition
  inversion stress
  Jansen
  jerk
  Johnson-Zuck-Wingate motor
  knee jerk reflex
  Lachman
  Lasègue
  MacIntosh lateral pivot shift
  McMurray
  Mills
  Morton
  Neer impingement
  Ninhydrin print
  Noyes flexion rotation drawer
  Ober
  patellar retraction
  Patrick
  Phalen

test (cont.)
  pivot-shift
  posterior drawer
  prone rectus
  quadriceps
  RA (rheumatoid arthritis)
  reverse pivot shift
  Romberg
  rotary instability
  saline acceptance
  Schirmer
  Schober
  Sherman block
  Silfverskiöld
  Simmonds
  skin resistance
  Slocum rotary instability test
  somatosensory
  sponge
  Spurling
  squat
  Stagnara wake-up
  station
  straight leg raising
  stress
  supine straight leg raising
  sweat
  Tensilon
  tensing
  Thomas
  thumbnail
  tourniquet
  Trendelenburg
  triceps jerk reflex
  triketohydrindene hydrate print
  varus stress
  Voshell
  wake-up
  Weber
  Wilson
  Wright-Adson
  Yeager
  Yergason
tester
  Cybex
  Jamar grip

testing, Doppler ultrasound segmental
　　blood pressure
tetanus prophylaxis
Teufel brace
Teuffer technique
Tevdek suture
TFA (tibiofemoral angle)
TFL (tensor fasciae latae)
THA (total hip arthroplasty)
Tharies hip replacement
Thatcher nail
thenar eminence
therapist
　　occupational
　　physical
therapy
　　conservative
　　occupational
　　physical
thermolabile plastic
Thiemann disease
Thiersch thin split free graft
thighbone
Thomas collar cervical orthosis
Thomas-Thompson-Straub transfer
　　technique
Thompson quadricepsplasty
Thompson telescoping V osteotomy
Thompson, F.R., endoprosthesis
Thompson-Epstein classification of
　　femoral fracture
Thompson-Henry technique
Thomsen disease
thoracic spine, T1 to T12
thoracic outlet syndrome
thoracolumbar spine
thoracotomy
thorax, thoraces, thoracic
Thornton bar; nail; plate; screw
THR (total hip replacement)
thrombin powder
thrombin-soaked Gelfoam
thumb
　　bowler's
　　Flotan
　　gamekeeper's

thumb *(cont.)*
　　spring swivel
　　trigger
thumb duplication, Wassel type IV
thumb-in-palm deformity
thumbnail test
thumb pinch power
thumb polydactyly, Wassel classifica-
　　tion of
Thurst plate femoral prosthesis
Thurston-Holland sign
Ti-6Al-4V implant metal
Ti-Thread prosthesis
tibia valga
tibia vara
tibial collateral ligament (TCL)
tibial plateau prosthesis
tibiofemoral angle (TFA)
tibiofibular syndesmosis
tibiotalar
tic
Ti-Con prosthesis
Tiemann nail
Tietze syndrome
tightener, wire
Tikhoff-Linberg shoulder resection
Tillaux fracture
Tillman prosthesis
tilt
　　angular
　　pelvic
　　talar
time
　　anesthesia
　　capillary filling
　　capillary refill
　　loading
　　operating
　　procedure
　　total tourniquet
　　tourniquet
　　warm ischemic
times (x)
tincture of belladonna
tincture of benzoin
tincture of time (TOT)

Tinel sign
tingle, tingling
tip of medial malleolus
tiring (cerclage)
tissue
    adipose
    bursal
    cartilaginous
    connective
    devitalized
    fatty
    fibrous
    granulation
    intervening connective
    muscular
    osseous
    periarticular
    periosteal
    revascularized
    scar
    skeletal
    soft
    subcutaneous
    viable
Titan hip prosthesis
titanium implant
titer
    ASO (antistreptolysin)
    B. burgdorferi (for Lyme disease)
Tivanium implant metal
TLSO (thoracolumbosacral orthosis)
    brace
Tobruk splint
toe, toes
    clawtoe
    downgoing
    great
    mallet
    marathoner's
    Morton
    set ankle of
    splaying of
    tennis
    upgoing
    webbed
toe box, high

toeing in
toeing out
toenail, ingrown
toe plate extension
    cast with dorsal
    cast with volar
toe walk(ing)
toggle
Tohen tendon technique
tomogram, tomography
tongs, traction
    Barton
    Barton-Cone
    Böhler
    cervical fracture
    Cherry
    Crutchfield-Raney
    Gardner-Wells
    Raney-Crutchfield
    sugar
    Trippi-Wells traction
    Vinke skull traction
tonus
tophaceous gout
tophi, gouty
tophus, tophi
Torg knee reconstruction
Torgerson-Leach modified technique
Tornwaldt bursitis
Toronto brace; splint
torque force
torque heel on shoe
torque load
torque, frictional
torsion, internal tibial (ITT)
torsion, tibial
torticollis (wryneck), congenital
torus fracture
TOT (tincture of time)
total hip replacement (THR)
total knee instrumentation, FIRST
total knee, PCA
Total Condylar Knee
touch sensation
touchdown weightbearing

tourniquet
  double
  Esmarch
  pneumatic
  TCPM pneumatic
tourniquet control, exsanguination
towel
  Charnley
  Huck
  sterile
Townley TARA prosthesis
Townsend-Gilfillan screw
trabecula, trabeculae, trabecular
tracing paper
track normally
track, tracked
Tracker knee brace
tracking, patellar
tract
traction
  Anderson
  axis
  Baker trabecular
  balanced skeletal
  Barton-Cone tong
  Bendixen-Kirschner
  Blackburn
  Böhler tong
  Bryant
  Buck
  cervical
  Cherry tong
  Cotrel
  Crego-McCarroll
  Crile head
  Crutchfield skeletal tong
  Dunlop
  elastic
  exo-static
  floating
  Freiberg
  Frejka
  Gallo
  Gardner-Wells tong
  gentle
  Granberry

traction *(cont.)*
  halo-femoral
  halo-pelvic
  halter
  Hamilton
  Handy-Buck
  Hare
  head-halter
  Hoke-Martin
  Jones suspension
  K wire skeletal
  Kessler
  Keys-Kirschner
  King cervical
  Kirschner skeletal
  Kuhlmann
  Logan
  longitudinal
  low-profile halo
  Lyman-Smith
  manual
  McBride tripod pin
  Neufeld
  Orr-Buck
  Ortho-Vent
  Pease-Thomson
  pelvic
  Perkins
  Pugh
  Raney-Crutchfield tong
  Roger Anderson
  rubber band
  Russell
  Sayre
  skeletal
  skin
  snug
  split Russell skeletal
  Steinmann
  sugar-tong
  suspension
  Syms
  three-point skeletal
  trabecular
  Vinke tong
  Watson-Jones

traction *(cont.)*
   well leg
   Wells
   Zimfoam splint
   traction application
   traction handle, Barton
   Tracto-halter training, gait
   transarticular pin
   transcapitate fracture-dislocation
   transcarpal amputation
   transcervical fracture
   transcondylar fracture
   transcutaneous electrical nerve stimulation (TENS)
   transcutaneous oxygen tension determination
   transection, step-cut
   transfer
      Baker lateral semitendinosus
      Barr tendon
      Bateman modification of Mayer
      free flap
      Green
      Huber abductor digiti quinti
      iliopsoas
      Littler-Cooley abductor digiti quinti
      Neviaser-Wilson-Gardner
      tendon
      toe-to-hand
   transfixing pin
   transfixion screw, Glass-Bessen
   transhamate fracture-dislocation
   transitional vertebra
   translocation, Baker
   transmalleolar
   transplant
      d'Aubigne patellar
      free vascularized bone
      pedicled
      whole bone
   transposition
      subfascial
      tendon
   transscaphoid perilunate dislocation
   transtriquetral fracture-dislocation
   trapdoor

trapezial area
trapeziodeltoid interval
Trapezoidal-28 (T-28) internal prosthesis
trapezoidal osteotomy
trauma, musculoskeletal
trauma, traumatic, traumatically
Trautman Locktite prosthetic hook
tray
   Denis Browne
   tibial
treatment for scoliosis, electrical surface stimulation
tremor
Trendelenburg gait; position
trephine [*trephination* — handwritten annotation]
   bone
   Castroviejo
   Phemister biopsy
Trethowan-Stamm-Simmonds-Menelaus-Haddad technique
Tri-Axial elbow prosthesis
Tri-Con prosthesis
Tri-Lock hip prosthesis
triad, O'Donoghue
trial component (see *prosthesis*)
trial fit
trial range of motion
trial reduction
trial seating
triangle
   cervical
   clavipectoral
   Codman
   Hardy-Joyce
   iliofemoral
   infraclavicular
   Kager
   Langenbeck
   metal measuring
   Middeldorpf
   Petit
   posterior
   sacral
   von Weber
   Ward

| triangular | 140 | twister |

*Tubi-Grip* (handwritten at top)

triangular defect
triangulating
triangulation technique for arthroscope
triaxial semiconstrained elbow prosthesis
triceps jerk reflex test
trifurcation
triketohydrindene hydrate print test
Trillat procedure
trimalleolar fracture
trimmer, motorized
Trinkle brace and adapter
tripartite muscle origin
triplane osteotomy
triple arthrodesis
triple diapering
triploscope
tripod cane
tripod, McBride
Trippi-Wells traction tongs
triquetral fracture
triquetrolunate dislocation
triradiate cartilage
trisomy 21
trispiked
trocar, T-handle
trochanter
    greater
    lesser
trochanter, trochanteric
trochlea
trochlear defect
trolley, Tupper
Tronzo classification of inter-trochanteric fracture
tropism, facet
trouble ascending and descending stairs
trough, bone
trousers, MAST (medical antishock)
Trumble arthrodesis
Tsuji laminaplasty
TTAP (threaded titanium acetabular prosthesis)
tube
    Adson suction
    chest

tube *(cont.)*
    Hemovac suction
    Jergesen
    suction
    vent
tubercle
    Gerdy
    Ghon
    Lister
    tibial
tuberculosis of the hip
tuberosity
    greater
    lesser
tubing
    Dakin
    medullary vent
TufStuf II cast tape
tuft, finger
Tuli heel cup
tumor
    brown (hyperparathyroidism)
    desmoid
    dumbbell
    Enneking stain of malignant soft tissue
    Ewing
    giant cell tumor
    glomus
    Hodgkin
    Schwann
tunnel
    carpal
    cubital
    fibro-osseous
    subsartorial
Tupman plate
Tupper trolley
Turco clubfoot release technique
turgor
turnbuckles
Turner pin
Turner syndrome
Turyn sign
Twin Cities Lo-Profile halo
twister, Shifrin wire

*Trunnion* (handwritten at bottom)

Tycron suture
tyloma

# U, u

U approach
U drapes
U-shaped retractor
U.S. retractor
UBC (Univ. of British Columbia) brace
UCB (unilateral calcaneal brace)
UCB (University of California, Berkeley) foot orthosis
UCB shoe insert
UCBl (Univ. of California Berkeley insert)
UCI ankle prosthesis
UCP compression plate
Uematsu shoulder arthrodesis
UHMWPE (ultrahigh molecular weight polyethylene)
ulcer
    decubitus
    stasis
    trophic
ulnarward
Ultra-Flex orthopedic bed
ultrahigh molecular weight polyethylene (UHMWPE)
uncovertebral joint
under direct vision
undersurface of patella
ungual tuberosity
unhappy triad of O'Donoghue
unicameral bone cyst
unicompartmental knee prosthesis
Unicondylar Geomedic Hemi-Knee system
union, delayed fracture
unit
    Bovie coagulating

unit *(cont.)*
    Hydra-Cadence gait-control
    musculotendinous
    TENS
Unitek steel crown
univalved
Universal hip prosthesis
Unna boot wrap
unopposed
UPF (universal proximal femur)
upgoing toes
Upper 7 head halter
upper limits of normal
urate crystal
uric acid crystal
Uslenghi plate
Utah artificial arm

# V, v

V blade plate
V capsulotomy
V medullary nail
V nail plate
V osteotomy, Japas
V-shaped incision
V-Y plasty
V-Y quadricepsplasty
Vac-Pac
vaginal ligament of hand
Valentine splint
valgus deformity
valgus instability
Valsalva maneuver
valsalva'd (coined past tense verb form)
Van Ness procedure
Vanghetti prosthesis
Vanzetti sign
varicosities, superficial
Varikopf hip prosthesis
Varney acromioclavicular brace

Varney pin
varus-valgus adjustment screw
vascular invasion
vascularity
Vastamäki paralysis
vastus lateralis muscle
vastus medialis advancement
 (VMA)
vastus medialis obliquus (VMO)
Velcro fitting; splint; strap
Veleanu-Rosianu-Ionescu technique
Velpeau bandage; cast
velum
Venable plate
Venable-Stuck nail; pin; screw
venography, intraosseous
Verbrugge clamp; needle
Verdan technique
Veress needle
Vernier caliper
verruca plantaris
version, internal and external
vertebra, vertebrae
 scalloping of
 transitional
 wedging of olisthetic
vertebra plana fracture
vertebrectomy, Bohlman anterior
 cervical
Vesely-Street nail; splint
vest
 halo
 Vitrathene
Vi-Drape
viability
Vibram rockerbottom shoe
vibration sensation
Vicryl figure-of-8 sutures
Victorian brace
Vidal-Ardrey modified Hoffman device
Vidicon vacuum chamber pickup tube
 for video camera (arthroscopy)
view (x-ray)
 AP
 apical
 apical lordotic

view *(cont.)*
 axial sesamoid
 axillary
 baseline
 Beath
 Böhler calcaneal
 Böhler lumbosacral
 Breuerton
 carpal tunnel
 Carter-Rowe
 cine
 coalition
 coned-down
 cross-table
 dens (cervical spine)
 dorsoplantar
 Dunlop-Shands
 Ferguson
 frogleg lateral
 Harris
 Harris-Beath
 Hughston
 infrapatellar (of knees)
 intraoperative
 inversion ankle stress
 Jones
 Jude pelvic
 lateral oblique
 mortise
 nonstanding lateral oblique
 notch
 oblique
 odontoid
 plantar axial
 push-pull ankle stress
 push-pull hip
 skijump
 skyline
 spot
 standing dorsoplantar
 standing lateral
 standing weightbearing
 sunrise
 sunset
 tangential
 true lateral

view *(cont.)*
  tunnel
  von Rosen
  Waters
  weightbearing dorsoplantar
Vigilon dressing
villonodular synovitis
villous synovitis
Vinertia implant metal
Vinke skull traction tongs
Virtullene brace material
vise, mechanic's pin
vision, under direct
Vistec x-ray detectable sponge
visualized
Vitallium implant metal
Vitallium Küntscher nail
Vitrathene vest
Viva shoes
VMA (vastus medialis advancement)
VMO (vastus medialis obliquus)
Vogue arm sling
volar wrist
volarly, volarward
Volkman rake retractor
Volkov-Oganesian external fixation
Volz wrist prosthesis
Volz-Turner reattachment technique
Vom Saal pin
vomer
von Bekhterev reflex
von Lackum transection shift jacket
von Langenbeck periosteal elevator
von Recklinghausen disease
von Rosen cruciform splint
von Schwann, law of
Voorhoeve disease
Voshell sign; test
Vostal classification of radial fracture
Vulpius-Compere gastrocnemius
  lengthening

# W, w

W-plasty
WACH (wedge adjustable cushioned
  heel) shoe
wad, flexor
wadding, cotton sheet
waddle, duck
Wadsworth unconstrained elbow
  prosthesis
Wagner modification of Syme
  amputation
Wagner retractor
Wagner-Schanz screw apparatus
Wagoner cervical technique
Wagstaffe fracture
Wainwright plate
waist of the phalanx
walk
  heel
  toe
walker
  four-point
  Rolator
  rubber wedge
walking
  heel
  heel and toe
  nonweightbearing crutch
  toe
Walldius knee prosthesis
Wangensteen needle holder
Ward triangle
Warm Springs brace
warmth, joint
Warner-Farber ankle fixation technique
Warren-Marshall classification
wart
Wartenberg sign
washer
  oval
  toothed
Wassel classification of thumb
  polydactyly
Wassel type IV thumb duplication

Watanabe classification of discoid
 meniscus
Watco brace
waterpick, waterpicked
Waters x-ray view
Watkins fusion technique
Watson-Cheyne technique
Watson-Jones fracture repair
Waugh knee prosthesis
wax, bone
WCS (Wisconsin Compression System)
weakness
 breakaway
 motor
wear-and-tear
weaver's bottom
Weaver-Dunn acromioclavicular
 technique
web
 finger
 thumb
Webb stove bolt
webbed toes
webbing of fingers
Weber-Brunner-Freuler-Boitzy
 technique
Weber-Vasey traction-absorption wiring
 technique
Webril bandage
Webster needle holder
Weck osteotome
wedge
 compensatory
 medial heel
 Yancy cast
wedging of olisthetic vertebra
weightbearing crutches
weightbearing with crutches
weightbearing
 partial
 progression to
 touchdown
weightbearing dome of acetabulum
weight-relieving calipers
weights and pulleys
Weil splint

Weiss spring
Weit-Arner retractor
Weitlaner retractor
Wells traction
Wenger plate
Werdnig-Hoffmann disease
Wertheim splint
West and Soto-Hall patella technique
Westfield acromioclavicular
 immobilizer
Westin tenodesis
Westin-Turco category
wheelchair, Amigo mechanical
whirlpool bath
White epiphysiodesis
Whitecloud-LaRocca cervical
 arthrodesis
Whiteside Ortholoc II condylar
 femoral prosthesis
Whitesides tissue pressure
 determination
Whitesides-Kelly cervical technique
whitlow, herpetic
Whitman femoral neck reconstruction
whole bone transplant
Wiberg, CE angle of
Wiberg type II patellar contour
wide toebox shoe
Wilke boot
Wilkins classification of radial fracture
William Harris hip prosthesis
Williams-Haddad technique
willow fracture
Wilmington jacket
Wilson-McKeever arthroplasty
Wilson procedure for extra-articular
 fusion of elbow
Wilson-Burstein (DF80) hip prosthesis
Wilson-Jacobs tibial fracture fixation
 technique
Wilson-Johansson-Barrington cone
 arthrodesis
Wilson-McKeever shoulder technique
Wiltberger anterior cervical approach
Wiltse osteotomy of ankle
Winberger line

wince, wincing
Windlass mechanism
window, cortical
wing of ilium
wing, iliac
Wingfield frame
Wink retractor
wink, anal
Winograd technique for ingrown nail
Winquist-Hansen classification of femoral fracture
Winter spondylolisthesis technique
wire, wiring
    Bunnell pullout
    calibrated guide
    circular
    compression
    Drummond
    Ilizarov
    interfragmentary
    K (Kirschner)
    Kirschner (K)
    Magnuson
    monofilament
    nonthreaded
    olive
    Oppenheimer spring
    Schauwecker patellar tension band
    sharp-pointed
    stainless steel
    Thiersch
    threaded
    unthreaded
wire crimper, Caparosa
Wirth-Jager tendon technique
Wisconsin Compression System (WCS)
Wissinger rod
Wolf arthroscope
Wolfe-Böhler cast breaker
Wolfe-Kawamoto bone graft
Wolff law
wood screw (woodscrew)
Woodward technique
wound
    closed
    exit

wound *(cont.)*
    gunshot
    incised
    open
    puncture
    stab
wrap
    Ace
    Coban
    gauze
    Kerlix
    neck
    Unna
    Unna boot
wrapping, stump
wrench
    Allen
    cannulated
    Fox
    Harrington flat
    hex
    Müller
    socket
Wright plate
Wright-Adson test
Wrisberg ligament
wrist
    volar
    Volz
wristdrop
wryneck (torticollis)

# X, x

x (times)
x-ray tray, Bucky
x-ray view (see *view*)
xanthoma, malignant fibrous
Xenophor femoral prosthesis
Xeroform gauze dressing
XIP (x-ray in plaster)
xiphoid process
XOP (x-ray out of plaster)

# Y, y

Y bone plate
Y fracture
Y line
Y osteotomy
Y plate
Y-shaped incision
Y-T fracture
Yale brace
Yancy cast wedge
Yeager test
Yee posterior shoulder approach
Yergason sign
Yergason test of shoulder subluxation
Yoke transposition procedure
Young hinged knee prosthesis
Young-Vitallium hinged prosthesis
Yount procedure
Yucca board

# Z, z

Z fixation nail
Z-plasty, Cozen-Brockway
Z-plasty incision
Z-plasty local flap graft
Z-plasty tenotomy
Z plate
Zahn, line of
Zancolli procedure for clawhand
    deformity
Zaricznyj ligament technique
Zarins-Rowe ligament technique
Zazepen-Gamidov technique
Zeier transfer technique
Zickel subtrochanteric fracture fixation
Zielke instrumentation for scoliosis
    spinal fusion
zigzag finger incision
Zim-Zap rib belt
Zimalite implant metal
Zimaloy implant metal
Zimfoam head halter
Zimmer Cibatome cement eater
Zimmer Osteo-Stim
Zimmer Y plate
Zimmerman pericyte
Zlotsky-Ballard classification of
    acromioclavicular injury
Zollinger leg holder
Zoroc plaster
Zucker splint
Zuelzer awl

# References

# Orthopedic References

## Orthopedics

Bennington, James L. *Saunders Dictionary & Encyclopedia of Laboratory Medicine and Technology.* Philadelphia: W. B. Saunders Co., 1984.

Blauvelt, Carolyn T., and Fred R. T. Nelson. *A Manual of Orthopaedic Terminology.* 3rd ed. St. Louis: C. V. Mosby Co., 1985.

*Campbell's Operative Orthopaedics.* 7th ed., 4 vols., edited by A. H. Crenshaw. St. Louis: C. V. Mosby, 1987.

Crowley, Leonard V. *Introduction to Human Disease.* 2nd ed. Boston: Jones and Bartlett Publishers, 1988.

Fuller, Joanna R. *Surgical Technology: Principles and Practice.* 2nd ed. Philadelphia: W. B. Saunders Co., 1986.

*The SUM Program Orthopedic Transcription Unit.* Modesto, Ca.: Health Professions Institute, 1988.

## General Medicine and Surgery

Billups, Norman F., and Shirley M. Billups. *American Drug Index.* 32nd ed. Philadelphia: J. B. Lippincott Co., 1988.

Campbell, Linda C. *The Anatomy Word Book.* Modesto, Ca.: Prima Vera Publications, 1989.

Chabner, Davi-Ellen. *The Language of Medicine,* 3rd ed. Philadelphia: W. B. Saunders Co., 1985.

*Dorland's Illustrated Medical Dictionary.* 27th ed. Philadelphia: W. B. Saunders Co., 1988.

Logan, Carolynn M., and M. Katherine Rice. *Logan's Medical and Scientific Abbreviations.* Philadelphia: J. B. Lippincott Co., 1987.

Lorenzini, Jean A. *A Medical Phrase Index.* Oradell, N.J.: Medical Economics Co., 1978.

*Melloni's Illustrated Medical Dictionary.* 2nd ed. Edited by Dox, Melloni, and Eisner. Baltimore: Williams & Wilkins Publishing Co., 1985.

*The Merck Manual.* 14th ed. Rahway, N.J.: Merck & Co., 1982.

Miller, Benjamin F., and Claire Brackman Keane. *Encyclopedia and Dictionary of Medicine, Nursing, and Allied Health.* 4th ed. Philadelphia: W. B. Saunders, 1987.

Pyle, Vera. *Current Medical Terminology.* 2nd ed. Modesto, Ca.: Prima Vera Publications, 1988.

Roe-Hafer, Ann. *The Medical & Health Sciences Word Book.* 2nd ed. Boston: Houghton-Mifflin, 1982.

Sloane, Sheila B. *Medical Abbreviations and Eponyms.* Philadelphia: W. B. Saunders, 1985.

Sloane, Sheila B. *The Medical Word Book.* 2nd ed. Philadelphia: W. B. Saunders Co., 1982.

*Stedman's Medical Dictionary.* 24th ed. Baltimore: Williams & Wilkins Co., 1982.

*Taber's Cyclopedic Medical Dictionary.* 15th ed. Ed. by Clayton L. Thomas. Philadelphia: F. A. Davis Co., 1985.

Taylor, Donna M., and Patricia A. Collins. *For Your Information.* Orange County Chapter, American Association for Medical Transcription, 1987.

Tessier, Claudia. *The Surgical Word Book.* Philadelphia: W. B. Saunders Co., 1981.

*Webster's Medical Desk Dictionary.* Springfield, Mass.: Merriam-Webster Inc., Publishers, 1986.

## Style, Grammar, Mechanics

*Chicago Manual of Style.* 13th ed. Chicago: The University of Chicago Press, 1982.

Diehl, Marcy O., and Marilyn T. Fordney. *Medical Typing and Transcribing: Techniques and Procedures.* 2nd ed. Philadelphia: W. B. Saunders Co., 1984.

Dirckx, John H., M.D. *The Language of Medicine: Its Evolution, Structure, and Dynamics.* 2nd ed. New York: Praeger Publishers, 1983.

Fowler, H. W. *A Dictionary of Modern English Usage.* 2nd ed. Rev. by Sir Ernest Gowers. New York: Oxford University Press, 1985.

Johnson, Edward D. *The Handbook of Good English.* New York: Facts on File Publications, 1982.

*Manual for Authors & Editors: Editorial Style & Manuscript Preparation.* 7th ed. Compiled for American Medical Association by William R. Barclay et al. Los Altos, Ca.: Lange Medical Publications, 1981.

Shertzer, Margaret. *The Elements of Grammar.* New York: Macmillan Publishing Co., 1986.

Tessier, Claudia, and Sally C. Pitman. *Style Guide for Medical Transcription.* Modesto, Ca.: American Association for Medical Transcription, 1985.

*Webster's Standard American Style Manual.* Springfield, Mass.: Merriam-Webster, Inc., Publishers, 1985.

*Words into Type.* Based on studies by Marjorie E. Skillin et al. 3rd ed. Englewood Cliffs, N.J.: Prentice-Hall, Inc., 1974.

## English Dictionaries

*The American Heritage Dictionary.* 2nd ed. New York: Houghton Mifflin, 1983.
*The New Lexicon Webster's Dictionary of the English Language.* New York: Lexicon Publications, Inc., 1987.
*Oxford American Dictionary.* Compiled by Eugene Ehrlich et al. New York: Oxford University Press, 1980.
*The Random House Dictionary of the English Language.* 2nd ed., Unabridged. Ed. by Flexner and Hauck. New York: Random House, 1987.
*Webster's Ninth New Collegiate Dictionary.* Springfield, Mass.: Merriam-Webster, Inc., 1983.